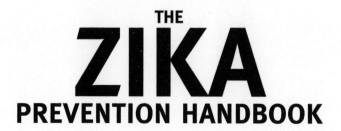

THE
ZIKA
PREVENTION HANDBOOK

THE ZIKA

PREVENTION HANDBOOK

EVERYTHING YOU NEED TO KNOW TO STAY SAFE

ALEXANDER WEBB

With a foreword by Laura D Kramer, PhD, FASTMH

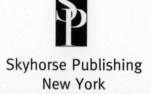

Skyhorse Publishing
New York

The information given in this volume is for educational and entertainment purposes only and does not constitute medical advice or the practice of medicine. No provider-patient relationship, explicit or implied, exists between the publisher, authors, and readers. This book does not substitute for such a relationship with a qualified provider. The strategies discussed in this volume are based on current knowledge; advances in our understanding of prevention, care, and treatment of Zika virus may change significantly in the future. The authors and publisher strongly urge their readers to seek modern and standard medical care with certified practitioners whenever and wherever it is available.

The reader should never delay seeking medical advice, disregard medical advice, or discontinue medical treatment because of information in this book or any resources cited in this book.

Although the authors have researched all sources to ensure accuracy, they assume no responsibility for errors, omissions, or other inconsistencies therein. Neither do the authors or publisher assume liability for any harm caused by the use or misuse of any methods, products, instructions, or information in this book or any resources cited in this book.

Skyhorse Publishing books may be purchased in bulk at special discounts for sales promotion, corporate gifts, fund-raising, or educational purposes. Special editions can also be created to specifications. For details, contact the Special Sales Department, Skyhorse Publishing, 307 West 36th Street, 11th Floor, New York, NY 10018 or info@skyhorsepublishing.com.

Skyhorse® and Skyhorse Publishing® are registered trademarks of Skyhorse Publishing, Inc.®, a Delaware corporation.

Visit our website at www.skyhorsepublishing.com.

10 9 8 7 6 5 4 3 2 1

Library of Congress Cataloging-in-Publication Data is available on file.

Cover design by Brian Peterson
Cover photo by iStockPhoto.com

Print ISBN: 978-1-5107-2220-0
Ebook ISBN: 978-1-5107-2221-7

Printed in the United States of America

Contents

Acknowledgements

Every book is a team effort, and I first would like to thank the team at Hollan Publishing, especially Holly Schmidt and Monica Sweeney, for their help, encouragement, and advice. Thanks are also due to the publisher, Skyhorse.

This book also owes a great debt to the men and women of the Centers for Disease Control and Prevention, who have issued great information and guidelines on the Zika virus, some of which is excerpted or adapted for this book. Their hard work is not only saving lives, but is also responsible for much of the information and content in this book.

Thanks are also due to Laura Kramer for her great foreword and for helping improve the text. I would also like to thank Hans Verkerke, who helped me clarify some issues that arose while writing the book.

As a writer, I have been extremely fortunate to receive extremely valuable advice, encouragement, and mentorship from John Thompson. I would also like to thank Amy Gary, who has supported my career and freely shared her detailed knowledge of the industry. I would also like to thank Nguyen An, Noah Davis, Tom Grundy, Kristin Wong, Stuart Thornton, and Isak Ladegaard for sharing their writing expertise with me.

All along I've been fortunate to have support and encouragement from my friends around the world, including (but certainly not limited to): Alan Gregory, Greg Leichner, Jeffrey Leung, Linda and Richard Barr, Mark Erhart, Matt Chambers, Patrick Bostrom, Peter Chan, Peter Farrell, Phillip Walker, Pratyush Rai, Rob Martin, Ryohei Mizusawa, Sonny Dhanda, Takuya Kon, Will

Massie, Zach Parks, KJ Yoo, the Spiekermann family, Pei Wang, and many, many, more.

I would also like to thank two teachers who have had a positive impact on my life, Baniel Cheung and Chris Bunin.

Finally, I would like to thank my family and relatives, including Vanessa and the entire Cao family, for all the love and support they have provided me over the years. That is truly the greatest gift of all.

Foreword

Zika virus is an arbovirus (arthropod-borne virus), which is a type of virus that passes most commonly between mosquitoes, sand flies, or ticks to humans and other species. Zika virus is carried by *Aedes aegypti* mosquitoes, the same species commonly associated with the spread of yellow fever, dengue, and chikungunya viruses. Not only are these viruses carried by the same mosquito, they have similar early symptoms in infected humans, making it difficult to diagnose which disease the patient has. Zika, however, while generally a mild illness, is particularly dangerous because it causes microcephaly and other neurologic disorders in babies infected in the womb. It also has been associated with increased numbers of cases in adults of Guillain-Barre syndrome, an autoimmune disorder affecting the peripheral nervous system following infection with a virus. Joint and ocular problems have been reported along with other abnormalities following Zika infection.

Zika virus is expanding its range at a rapid pace, which is having major global consequences. Currently in the summer of 2016, Zika virus is causing increasing numbers of cases in Florida, and appears to be spreading to other states such as Texas, and countries such as Taiwan, through viremic travelers.

It is not a question of whether a new arbovirus like Zika will emerge, but rather what will the new disease be, and when it will happen. In retrospect, we should have been able to predict the emergence of most of the mosquito-borne viruses that have come our way. In the past, viruses such as West Nile and dengue were not regarded as threats until they reached the US In fact, most people in the US had never even heard of West Nile virus! After West Nile arrived to fertile ground in New York in 1999, the virus flourished and spread from the east to west coast in approximately three years. Similarly, dengue has been increasing as a problem for the Americas. Over 2.5 billion people, greater than 30 percent of the world's population, in over 100 countries are at risk of dengue infection. There are annually scattered cases in the US, with an outbreak in Florida in 2009–2010. There is concern that climate warming may contribute to the expansion of the vector's range, and consequently, increasing numbers of cases.

Why are we seeing emergence of a growing number of viruses with serious medical consequences? The factors leading to this trend are many, including socio-economic, environmental, and ecological. The globalization of goods, rapid international travel by large numbers of people, and destruction of habitat bring humans into close contact with viruses. Land use changes such as urbanization, agricultural, and deforestation have significant impact on vector-borne disease. One example of this is the clearing of forests to build roads and houses, which brings down canopy-dwelling mosquitoes that normally would feed on non-human primates in the tree tops but, with cutting down trees, feed on humans at ground level. Furthermore, such destructive activities create new habitats for vectors, such as pools of water for mosquito breeding. Patterns of malaria and yellow fever, for example among others, have been affected by deforestation. What's more, urban crowding with inadequate infrastructure to support the growing population, lack of clean drinking water, poor water storage, ineffective mosquito control, and lack of approved, safe vaccines and therapeutics can all contribute to the increased spread of viruses like Zika.

Zika virus emergence in the Americas is a classic emergence event. The virus historically cycled in the Ugandan forest, after which it was named, between nonhuman primates and sylvatic mosquitoes. Humans became infected, but symptoms were largely mild or absent. The virus was then introduced into the Asian Pacific region where it diverged genetically significantly to form a separate lineage. The traffic of travelers and commercial goods between that region and the Americas is very high, and as a result, Zika virus was inadvertently introduced to Brazil. There the environment and population were very receptive to this new virus, where there was no previous exposure to Zika virus, where homes without mosquito-blocking screens are prevalent, where open water storage containers around homes act as breeding-grounds for mosquitoes, and where large sporting events with travelers attending from all over the world are common.

The biology and behavioral characteristics of *A. aegypti* make it an especially treacherous mosquito. After having emerged from the forests of Africa, this mosquito adapted itself extremely well to living in close proximity to humans, in part by laying eggs in water storage containers around homes. Mosquitoes emerge from these breeding grounds, mate, and have easy access to humans living in the surrounding area. Female mosquitoes will commonly feed more than once before laying each batch of eggs, meaning that each Zika virus-infected female can infect multiple people in a household. Also contributing to their success is that their eggs can dry and still survive, which means that they can withstand drought conditions and also be easily transported. There has been a resurgence of *A. aegypti* populations after having been eliminated in Brazil in 1955 and subsequently from most of the Americas. This was the result of a continental campaign initiated in 1916 by the Rockefeller

Foundation and followed up by the Pan American Health Organization in 1940–1960.

The combination of factors that lead to the emergence of mosquito-borne viruses make viruses such as Zika extremely difficult to control. A single viremic traveler can transport the virus anywhere she or he travels and establish infection in a new population. Novel control methods, while promising in the laboratory, have been less successful in the field for large-scale control. New Zika vaccines are in early trial. Rapid diagnostics are being developed. An integrated approach is clearly necessary, including vector control, improvement of basic public health infrastructure, vaccines, and antivirals. Each of these efforts requires significant federal, state, and local support and a strong base of basic research. *The Zika Prevention Handbook* will address much of what we have learned about Zika, explore unanswered questions, and propose directions we need to go. The reader can use the information provided to help protect themselves and consequently their neighbors, and to do their part to help prevent the virus's spread if they live in or are traveling to Zika virus-affected areas.

—Laura D Kramer, PhD, FASTMH

Introduction

In early 2015, Brazil faced 7,000 cases of a mystery virus—an illness with symptoms including fever, joint pain, and, above all, strange skin rashes. Authorities searched for the usual suspects, running tests for chikungunya, enterovirus, measles, and more, but they were all ruled out. Just what was infecting these people? It was Zika—but nobody knew that yet. In fact, they didn't even think to test for it because the virus was so obscure.

Just one year later, hundreds of thousands of people were infected, and Zika had spread to nearly every country in Latin America and the Caribbean. Birth defects spiked in the infected areas, and a worrying link between Zika and Guillain-Barré syndrome, which causes temporary paralysis, was becoming clear. Although Latin America was hit the hardest, it was already a global problem. Travelers who got the virus on vacation had brought it back to countries like Taiwan and South Korea.

In the span of a single year, Zika transformed from a mere footnote in virology textbooks into a household name with hundreds of thousands of confirmed cases. But how did this once-minor virus sneak up on the entire world? The story starts nearly seventy years ago.

In 1947, a new virus was discovered in a caged rhesus macaque monkey in Uganda's Zika Forest. In 1948, the same virus was again found nearby, this time in a mosquito, and the virus was given its now-famous name. For the next sixty years, the virus was obscure, infecting few people and making no headlines when it did. Zika's correlation with birth defects and temporary paralysis was unknown, and the virus was essentially forgotten.

It wasn't until 2007 that the first known Zika outbreak took place. Interestingly enough, it took place on Yap Island in Micronesia, a remote country in the Pacific Ocean. Around 70 percent of the residents of the island were infected, making it a huge and surprising outbreak. While this was major news to locals, in the rest of the world, this incident was hardly even reported. Zika remained a niche virus with minor effects. Part of the reason it escaped scrutiny is that the worst effects of the current outbreak—birth defects and paralysis—were not reported as occurring in the 2007 outbreak. Given Micronesia's distance from the rest of the world, Zika remained a footnote.

In 2013 and 2014, more Pacific islands began to suffer large numbers of Zika infections. From French Polynesia to Easter Island, multiple outbreaks occurred concurrent with increases in Guillain-Barré syndrome, providing the first evidence that Zika might be correlated to neurological problems.

By 2015, the focus had moved to South America, where Brazil was facing a looming health crisis. After initial confusion and questions over the mysterious outbreak in the country's northeast in May of 2015, the National Reference Laboratory of Brazil reported that Zika was the culprit. Most observers asked themselves, "What's Zika?"

Indeed, Zika has attracted so much attention not only because of its sudden, rapid spread, but also because of the mystery that continues to surround it. Although Zika is a mosquito-borne virus, it is not a normal one. Tom Frieden, director of the CDC, noted, "We've never before had a mosquito-borne disease that can cause a birth defect." To make matters worse, Zika can not only result in microcephaly—abnormally small heads in babies—but also spreads through sexual contact, presenting risks for women who want to conceive. And although the most well-known effects of Zika are birth defects, it is also correlated with Guillain-Barré syndrome, which can cause muscle weakness and even temporary paralysis.

Although scientists are racing to find a vaccine, for now Zika continues to spread. Thousands of babies around the world have been born with microcephaly, and fears over the virus caused several top athletes to skip the 2016 Olympics in Rio de Janeiro. Although Zika had long seemed like a faraway threat restricted to Latin America and Puerto Rico, on August 1, 2016, the CDC announced that Zika had been found in the Wynwood neighborhood of Miami, and advised against travel to the area. A few weeks later, Zika was also found in Miami Beach. This ushered in a new era of uncertainty for Americans, who were now left to wonder, "Am I next?"

This book is designed to answer all the questions you have about Zika—and hopefully some questions you haven't thought about yet. It covers everything from avoiding mosquitoes, to foreign travel, to sexual safety, to treating the symptoms of the virus. Although it is packed with information, nothing can replace a careful consultation with a healthcare professional. If you think you or your loved ones may have Zika, this book can serve as a guide. However, you should be sure to discuss your treatment options with a qualified professional armed with the latest information. Research continues to uncover new information about Zika, and treatment options, recommendations, and best practices may change over time.

1

About Zika

WHAT IS ZIKA?

Zika is a virus primarily spread by mosquitoes that can cause birth defects, temporary paralysis, and mild flulike symptoms. It is closely related to other serious viruses such as yellow fever, dengue, and Japanese encephalitis. Those at greatest risk from Zika are pregnant mothers and their unborn children, who may suffer birth defects, although all humans are susceptible to Zika. In a few cases, those affected by Zika may suffer from the rare Guillain-Barré syndrome (GBS), which can cause temporary or permanent paralysis.

Zika is a virus and a disease

Zika is both a virus and a disease. The Zika virus causes Zika fever, also known as Zika virus disease. In common usage, both the virus and the disease are called Zika. To keep things understandable, we will also follow this naming scheme.

What are its effects? How does it spread?

Zika is spread through numbers of mosquito species, but in the Americas, the important species are *Aedes aegypti* and *Aedes albopictus* mosquitoes, which are commonly referred to as the yellow fever and Asian tiger mosquitos, respectively. These mosquitos are present in many tropical and subtropical climates around the world. Most US states have a yellow fever or Asian tiger mosquito presence for at least some of the year. Zika has limited but serious effects. Although pregnant women and their unborn children face the most risk from the virus, adults are also vulnerable to Guillain-Barré syndrome (GBS), which can cause temporary or permanent paralysis. The CDC notes:

Zika can cause serious birth defects in babies born to women who were infected with Zika virus during pregnancy during pregnancy, especially those infected in the first trimester. Current CDC research suggests that Zika also is strongly associated with Guillain-Barré syndrome, a rare disorder that can cause muscle weakness and paralysis for a few weeks to several months. Only a small proportion of people with recent Zika virus infection get GBS. Most people fully recover from GBS, but some have permanent damage.

Zika can also spread through sex. People with Zika can pass the virus to their partners even if they do not have symptoms at the time, or if their symptoms have gone away. We do not know how long a person who has had Zika can pass it on through sex, although in one case it has been found in semen at least six months after infection. The mosquitoes that spread Zika usually do not live at elevations above 6,500 feet (2,000 meters). People who live in areas above this elevation are at a very low risk of getting Zika from a mosquito unless they visit or travel through areas of lower elevation. Because there is no vaccine or treatment for Zika, people living in areas with Zika should take steps to prevent infection.

HISTORY OF ZIKA

Zika got its name from Uganda's Zika Forest, where it was first isolated in 1947. Although scientists have known about the virus for more than fifty years, it was largely ignored, as it seemingly infected merely small numbers of people with minimal consequences. In 2007, the first known outbreak occurred on Yap Island in the Federated States of Micronesia, where an estimated 73 percent of residents aged three and above became infected.[1] After a few years of quiet, there were an estimated 19,000 cases in 2013 on French Polynesia, shortly followed by a 2014 outbreak on Easter Island.[2] Although there were multiple outbreaks in different locations over several years, Zika was still seen as an obscure virus that was only afflicting remote, sparsely populated locations.

The 2015 outbreak in Brazil changed that.

Multiple outbreaks of the virus quickly spread, infecting thousands in Brazil, Colombia, and across South America, Central America, and the Caribbean. Cases of microcephaly spiked, leading to more than 1,800 Brazilian babies with impaired development. Slow responses by several governments and uncertainty over the long-term effects of the virus meant that Zika began to enter the public consciousness, making headlines, dominating social media, and gathering attention around the globe. By summer 2016, the first locally transmitted cases were identified in Miami, adding the United States to the list of countries with local mosquito-borne transmission of the virus, and making many Americans wonder, "What is Zika and how can I protect myself?"

REPORTED CASES

WORLDWIDE

Since only around 20 percent of people with Zika actively experience symptoms of the virus, determining the total number of infected individuals is tough. Adding to the problem is the fact that this is a worldwide epidemic taking place in many countries, some of which have low-quality healthcare systems.

So far, Brazil has around 100,000 confirmed cases of Zika in 2016. The actual number of infected Brazilians is likely to be higher, as most infected people do not show symptoms of the disease. Colombia also has around 100,000 Zika cases in 2016, although as with Brazil, the real number of infected persons may be quite a bit higher. In Brazil there have been more than 1,800 cases of microcephaly during the epidemic.

Assuming that these numbers represent only infected people who have displayed symptoms, it is reasonable to estimate that well over a million people worldwide have contracted the virus. The US Surgeon General has estimated that Puerto Rico alone will have 875,000 cases by the end of 2016, making it likely that the true number of infected people worldwide is, or will soon be, in the multiple millions. Indeed the WHO has estimated that around three to four million people are likely to be infected by the end of 2016. These numbers may grow substantially over the years. One study estimates that around 2.2 billion people worldwide are at risk of contracting the virus.

USA

With over 10,000 confirmed cases in Puerto Rico, the Obama administration declared a public health emergency on August 12, 2016. Around 10 percent of these Puerto Rican cases involve pregnant women, the group most at risk from the Zika virus.

The actual number of Puerto Rican Zika cases is believed to be substantially higher because around 80 percent of people infected with Zika report no symptoms. Most of these people probably don't even know they are infected. The Surgeon General estimated that one-fourth of people in Puerto Rico will be infected with Zika by the end of 2016.[3] Given that the island has a population of 3.5 million, that means there is a potential for 875,000 cases by year end.

The virus has also been spread by local mosquitoes in American Samoa and the US Virgin Islands. While the virus is not yet spreading locally in Hawaii, there are worries that it could take hold, given that it is home to the same mosquitoes that spread dengue fever.

Most of the incidence of Zika in the continental US has been due to travelers returning home from trips to infected areas. Thus, nearly every US state has at least once infected resident. These people can potentially spread the virus through sexual contact, so it is very important to practice safe sex if you or your partner have potentially been exposed to Zika. This is covered in detail later in the book.

While current numbers of infections are low, the prevalence of Zika in the United States is likely to increase as local transmission cases rise. Florida has already experienced limited numbers of local transmission through mosquitoes. It is quite possible that the virus will become endemic to Florida and other southern portions of the US that provide a suitable habitat for the *Aedes* mosquitoes. In Texas, one baby whose mother got Zika while traveling died due to microcephaly. Cases like this may become more common as the virus spreads.

EXPECTED RANGE OF SPREAD

Zika is primarily spread by the *Aedes* species mosquitoes, which can only survive for part of the year in many parts of the United States. Except for people living in southern Florida, Puerto Rico, and other select warm areas of the U.S, Zika transmission should be essentially nonexistent in the colder months, and may not happen even in the summer.

The mosquitoes that can carry Zika have found in many states, including Alabama, Arizona, Arkansas, California,

Colorado, Connecticut, Delaware, Florida, Georgia, Hawaii, Illinois, Indiana, Iowa, Kansas, Kentucky, Louisiana, Maine, Maryland, Massachusetts, Minnesota, Mississippi, Missouri, Nevada, New Hampshire, New Jersey, Nebraska, New Mexico, New York, North Carolina, Ohio, Oklahoma, Pennsylvania, Rhode Island, South Carolina, Tennessee, Texas, Utah, Vermont, Virginia, West Virginia, and Wisconsin. However, many of the more northern states only have the potential for a relevant mosquito presence during peak summer temperatures.

The only states where these mosquitoes are not found are: Alaska, Idaho, Michigan, Montana, North Dakota, Oregon, South Dakota, Washington, and Wyoming.

Even those who live in warm climates can reduce their risk by taking the appropriate precautions regarding mosquitoes, including wearing clothing that covers more of the body, using mosquito repellent and sprays, and taking care to avoid mosquito-heavy areas.

While mosquitoes have geographic limitations, the sexual spread of Zika is theoretically unlimited. If you or your sexual partner has traveled to a Zika-prone area, or been exposed to the virus through other means, you may be at risk regardless of your geographic location.

ZIKA FAQ

Zika is a virus that recently broke into the public consciousness. If you're reading this book, you're worried about the effects of the virus and how it could affect you or your family. Zika is a serious disease, but one that has a limited scope. While the initial symptoms are generally minor, it can pose a serious risk to unborn children, and can, in rare cases, lead to Guillain-Barré syndrome (GBS), a disorder which can result in muscle weakness or paralysis.

New scientific research is being conducted every day, and our understanding of the virus continues to grow. To help us understand the current risks, causes, and situation resolving Zika, the CDC has created a FAQ to help you and your family understand the risks that Zika poses:

How do people get infected with Zika?

Zika is spread to people primarily through the bite of an infected *Aedes* species mosquito (*Aedes aegypti* and *Aedes albopictus*). A pregnant woman can pass Zika to her fetus during pregnancy or around the time of birth. Also, a person with Zika can pass it to his or her sex partners. [It is important] for people who have traveled to or live in places with Zika to protect themselves by preventing mosquito bites and sexual transmission of Zika.

What health problems can result from getting Zika?

Many people infected with Zika will have no symptoms, or mild symptoms that last several days to a week. However, Zika infection during pregnancy can cause a serious birth defect called microcephaly and other severe fetal brain defects. Guillain-Barré syndrome (GBS), an uncommon sickness of the nervous system, is also very likely triggered by Zika in a small number of cases.

Once someone has been infected with Zika, it's very likely they'll be protected from future infections. There is no evidence that past Zika infection poses an increased risk of birth defects in future pregnancies.

Should pregnant women travel to areas where Zika has been confirmed?

No. Pregnant women should not travel to any area with Zika. Travelers who go to places with outbreaks of Zika can be infected with Zika, and Zika infection during pregnancy can cause microcephaly and other severe fetal brain defects.

If I am traveling to an area with Zika, should I be concerned about Zika?

Travelers who go to places with Zika can be infected with Zika, and the CDC has issued travel notices for people traveling to those areas. Many people will have mild or no symptoms. However, Zika can cause microcephaly and other severe birth defects. For this reason, pregnant women should not travel to any area with Zika, and women trying to get pregnant should talk to their doctors before traveling or before their male partners travel. It is especially important that women who wish to delay or avoid pregnancy consistently use the most effective method of birth control that they are able to use. Those traveling to areas with Zika should take steps during and after they travel to prevent mosquito bites and sexual transmission of Zika.

What can people do to prevent Zika?

The best way to prevent Zika is to protect yourself and your family from mosquito bites:

- Use Environmental Protection Agency (EPA)-registered insect repellents.
- Wear long-sleeved shirts and long pants.
- Sleep under a mosquito bed net if air conditioned or screened rooms are not available, or if sleeping outdoors.
- Zika can be spread by a person infected with Zika to his or her sex partners. People whose partners have traveled to or live in an area with Zika can prevent Zika by using condoms (or other barriers that protect against infection) every time they have sex or by not having sex.

What are the symptoms of Zika virus disease?

The most common symptoms of Zika virus disease are fever, rash, joint pain, and red eyes. Other symptoms include muscle pain and headache. Many people infected with Zika won't have symptoms or will have mild symptoms, which can last for several days to a week.

How is Zika diagnosed?

To diagnose Zika, your doctor will ask you about recent travel and symptoms you may have, and collect blood or urine to test for Zika or similar viruses.

Can someone who returned from an area with Zika get tested for the virus?

Zika virus testing is performed at CDC and some state and territorial health departments. See your doctor if you have Zika symptoms and have recently visited an area with Zika. Your doctor may order tests to look for Zika or similar viruses like dengue and chikungunya.

What should pregnant women who have recently traveled to an area with Zika do?

Pregnant women who have recently traveled to an area with Zika should talk to their doctor about their travel, even if they don't feel sick. Pregnant women should see a doctor if they have any Zika symptoms during their trip or within two weeks after traveling. All pregnant women can protect themselves by avoiding travel to an area with Zika, preventing mosquito bites, and following recommended precautions against getting Zika through sex.

WHAT IS BEING DONE
ABOUT THE ZIKA EPIDEMIC?

The worldwide Zika epidemic has led to a surge in research and new efforts to fight the virus. Many scientists are working to develop a vaccine for the Zika virus, while others are trying to determine the link between Zika and Guillain-Barré syndrome. Given the severity of the problem, other less conventional methods, such as the use and deployment of genetically modified (GM) mosquitoes, are also being tried.

Vaccines

Multiple vaccines are currently in development and research is taking place around the world. On August 4, 2016, researchers working at the Walter Reed Army Institute of Research and Harvard's Beth Israel Hospital reported a breakthrough which some believe will lead to the first safe and effective Zika vaccine for humans.[4] All three of their vaccine test candidates were found safe and effective in monkeys. One of the potential vaccines under development, known as the ZPIV vaccine, will progress to human trials that should start in October of 2016.

Given that there are multiple vaccine candidates showing potentially strong effectiveness against the virus, many believe that an effective vaccine will be found. Be sure to check for the latest in vaccine news by visiting cdc.gov/zika.

Genetically modified mosquitoes

Oxitec, a British company, has released a genetically modified (GM) mosquito in parts of Brazil in cooperation with the local government. This GM mosquito is modified to sire progeny that are unable to successfully develop. Thus, any mosquitoes that mate with it will fail to produce viable offspring. According to

Oxitec, trials in Brazil, Panama, and the Cayman Islands have resulted in a "greater than 90 percent suppression of the wild *Ae. aegypti* mosquito population."[5] This is a large decline, especially given mosquitoes are often hard to fight in Brazil's humid and wet rainforest climate, but it requires release of very large numbers of GM mosquitoes.

Although these tests suggest this method is highly effective at controlling the mosquito population, some critics have argued that not enough is known about genetic modification and that there could be unintended consequences. Despite these fears, many scientists believe the use of GM mosquitoes may be necessary to control the spread of Zika. If GM technology is indeed safe when used in the wild, it represents a major breakthrough in the fight against mosquitoes and mosquito-borne illnesses.

CDC actions

The CDC has publicly described the steps and activities it is taking to keep the public safe:

- Developing laboratory tests to diagnose Zika
- Conducting studies to learn more about the link between Zika and microcephaly and Guillain-Barré syndrome
- Monitoring and reporting cases of Zika, which will help improve our understanding of how and where Zika is spreading
- Providing guidance to travelers and Americans living in areas with current outbreaks
- Surveillance for the virus in the United States, including US territories
- Supporting on the ground in areas with Zika

- Conducting a study to evaluate the persistence of Zika virus in semen and urine among male residents of the United States.

Public Health Emergency in Puerto Rico

On August 12, 2016, the Obama administration declared a public health emergency in Puerto Rico due to the Zika epidemic sweeping the US territory. This declaration will enable Puerto Rico to obtain the resources it needs to continue fighting Zika.

Secretary of Health and Human Services Sylvia Mathews Burwell declared the emergency and said, "This Administration is committed to meeting the Zika outbreak in Puerto Rico with the necessary urgency." She added, "As the first virus that can be transmitted by mosquitoes known to cause severe birth defects, we are working closely with Puerto Rican officials to pursue solutions to fight the virus in Puerto Rico with a focus on protecting pregnant women and continuing our efforts with jurisdictions throughout the United States to address this public health threat. This emergency declaration allows us to provide additional support to the Puerto Rican government and reminds us of the importance of pregnant women, women of childbearing age, and their partners taking additional steps to protect themselves and their families from Zika."

The governor of Puerto Rico, Alejandro Garcia Padilla, said, "The threat of Zika to future generations of Puerto Ricans is evident, and I feel a responsibility to do everything that is within my reach to make sure we fight the spread of the virus. This is why we are actively looking for alternatives to prevent the number of infections from increasing. The declaration made by HHS, which grants access to certain funds, is another example of collaboration between the federal government and the government of Puerto Rico. We will continue our campaign to guide Puerto Ricans on the steps needed to prevent becoming infected with Zika; especially to prevent the virus from affecting pregnant women. We will also continue assisting communities on the island in order to eliminate potential breeding sites and using land methods to attack adult mosquitoes. I want to reemphasize the importance that citizens have in actively participating alongside the authorities in prevention efforts against the virus."

Puerto Rico is the center of the Zika epidemic in the United States, so it is crucial that the US and Puerto Rican governments work together to solve this crisis. This order is a step in the right direction and signals that both governments are taking the problem seriously.

ZIKA: EPIDEMIC VS. ENDEMIC

Epidemic and endemic are two commonly misunderstood words used to describe the spread of a disease. Epidemic sounds like a scary word, but it is really just means a country is experiencing outbreaks of Zika at a level higher than normal. On a contrary, a virus that is endemic to the country is present and infecting people, but not spreading at a higher-than-usual rate. The CDC has created a FAQ which breaks down the situation:

What does it mean when you say that a country has "endemic Zika"?

In some countries, there is evidence that Zika has existed there for years, and the countries may occasionally report new cases. A large number of local residents of these countries may be immune to Zika, so occasional cases may occur but generally do not become outbreaks. In these countries, the virus does not spread as quickly as in countries where it is newly introduced.

What is the risk of getting Zika in a country with endemic Zika?

We do not know the risk of getting Zika in a country with endemic Zika, but we think it is lower than in countries with epidemic Zika. Although the risk is likely to be low, it is not zero.

Why aren't you posting travel notices for countries with endemic Zika?

CDC does not post travel notices for diseases that have existed in a place for years (endemic diseases), unless the number of cases rises to the level of an outbreak. Although we do not know the risk of getting Zika in a country with endemic Zika, we think it is lower than in countries with epidemic Zika. In countries with epidemic Zika, the outbreak spreads quickly, and the risk to travelers is higher.

When would you post a travel notice for a country with endemic Zika?

We would post a travel notice for a country with endemic Zika if there were a sudden increase in the number of cases. The Zika situation is evolving, and recommendations may change as we learn more about the risk to travelers.

Why does the outbreak spread quickly in a country with epidemic Zika?

In the Americas, where Zika was newly introduced, it spread quickly because the local population was not immune. A population only becomes immune after a substantial proportion of people have been infected with the virus.

Will countries with newly introduced Zika become countries with endemic Zika?

This is likely. We cannot say for sure how long it will take, but it is likely to be years. As the local population becomes immune, spread of Zika will slow, and these countries will move to the list of endemic countries. When this happens, the travel notices will be taken down. However, it is possible that a country could experience another outbreak, in which case a new travel notice will be posted.

Is it safe for pregnant women to travel to countries with endemic Zika?

Although the risk of getting Zika in countries with endemic Zika is likely lower than in countries with epidemic Zika, it is not zero. Therefore, there is still a risk that a pregnant woman could get Zika and pass it to her fetus. Pregnant women or women who are planning to become pregnant should discuss their travel plans with their doctor. If they choose to travel, they should strictly follow steps to prevent mosquito bites.

Is it safe for women who are not pregnant and men to travel to countries with epidemic Zika?

Many people infected with Zika will not have symptoms or will only have mild symptoms, such as fever, rash, joint pain, and conjunctivitis (red eyes). However, infection during pregnancy can cause severe birth defects in a developing fetus.

Women and men who are considering getting pregnant should discuss their plans with their doctor. If they choose to travel, they should strictly follow steps to prevent mosquito bites.

If I take precautions to prevent mosquito bites, is it safe for me to travel to a country with endemic Zika?

Because Zika is mainly spread by mosquito bites, preventing mosquito bites will help prevent Zika. Because Zika can also be spread through sex, you should also not have unprotected sex with anyone who lives in or has recently traveled to a country with endemic Zika.

Could Zika become epidemic or endemic in the United States?

There may be small outbreaks of Zika in parts of the United States, but we think it is very unlikely Zika will become epidemic or endemic. Visit the CDC site for the latest information on Zika in the United States. The mosquitoes that spread Zika are mainly found in the southern United States, and there are very few areas that stay warm enough all year for the mosquitoes to survive through the winter. In addition, air conditioning and window and door screens are commonly used, so people in the United States are not as exposed to mosquitoes as are people in many other areas.

2

Where is it?

If you want to protect yourself from Zika, you first need to know where it is. Unfortunately, Zika is a worldwide threat, but currently most prevalent in South America, particularly in Brazil. Parts of the United States like Puerto Rico and Florida have also been hit by local transmission of the virus. We have included detailed coverage of Brazil, Puerto Rico, and Florida, in addition to broad coverage of all infected locations.

TRAVEL ADVISORIES

The CDC issued travel advisories for many countries suffering from Zika virus outbreaks. This list is constantly changing, so be sure to check out cdc.gov/zika for the most updated information. As of August 2016, the CDC has issued travel notices or advisories for these countries/areas:

Africa:
Cape Verde

North America:
Mexico; Miami-Dade County, Florida.

The Caribbean
Anguilla, Antigua and Barbuda, Aruba, Barbados, Bonaire, Cayman Islands, Cuba, Curaçao, Dominica, Dominican Republic, Grenada, Guadeloupe, Haiti, Jamaica, Martinique, the

Commonwealth of Puerto Rico, Saba, Saint Barthelemy, Saint Lucia, Saint Martin, Saint Vincent and the Grenadines, Sint Eustatius, Sint Maarten, Trinidad and Tobago, Turks and Caicos Islands, US Virgin Islands

Central America
Belize, Costa Rica, El Salvador, Guatemala, Honduras, Nicaragua, Panama

The Pacific Islands
American Samoa, Fiji, Marshall Islands, Micronesia, New Caledonia, Papua New Guinea, Samoa, Tonga

South America
Argentina, Bolivia, Brazil, Colombia, Ecuador, French Guiana, Guyana, Paraguay, Peru, Suriname, Venezuela

PRECAUTIONARY MEASURES WHILE TRAVELING

What can travelers do to prevent Zika?
Since there is no cure for Zika, your most important line of defense is preventing getting bitten by mosquitoes. Wearing long-sleeved clothing, using a proper mosquito repellent, and taking other steps to prevent getting a bite in the first place will go a long way towards preventing the spread of the virus. The CDC notes:

There is no vaccine or medicine for Zika. Travelers can protect themselves by preventing mosquito bites:

- Cover exposed skin by wearing long-sleeved shirts and long pants. Use EPA-registered insect repellents containing DEET, picaridin, oil of lemon eucalyptus (OLE, also called para-menthane-diol [PMD]), or IR3535. Always use as directed.

- Pregnant and breastfeeding women can use all EPA-registered insect repellents, including DEET, according to the product label.
- Most repellents, including DEET, can be used on children older than two months. (OLE should not be used on children younger than three years.)
- Use permethrin-treated clothing and gear (such as boots, pants, socks, and tents). You can buy pre-treated clothing and gear or treat them yourself.
- Stay in places with air conditioning and window and door screens to keep mosquitoes outside.
- Sleep under a mosquito bed net if air conditioned or screened rooms are not available or if sleeping outdoors.
- Mosquito netting can be used to cover babies younger than two months old in carriers, strollers, or cribs to protect them from mosquito bites.
- Because Zika can be sexually transmitted, if you have sex (vaginal, anal, or oral) while traveling, you should use condoms.

Given the risk of sexual transmission of Zika, practicing safe sex is key. If you or your partner is traveling to an infected area, you must not only protect yourself from mosquitoes but also from the sexual transmission of the virus. Since Zika has been found in semen as long as six months after infection, you should be sure to ask your partner about their extended travel history to ensure they are not likely to carry the Zika virus.

If you are likely to engage in sexual activity in an infected area, be sure to use condoms or other blocking contraceptives.

Be aware that contraceptives may not always be easily available in certain foreign countries, and that bringing your own before you travel is wise. Further information on contraceptives and the sexual transmission of Zika is covered later in this book.

BRAZIL

Overview

Brazil is one of the world's great countries, famous for samba, amazing beaches, incredible food, and a fascinating, diverse culture. Sadly, it has recently been in the news for other reasons—namely, Zika. The current Zika epidemic started in Brazil, and thus much of the world's attention has been on this South American country. Although Brazil is widely seen as the epicenter of the current Zika epidemic, travel is possible if appropriate steps are taken. However, there are important exceptions. The CDC currently recommends that women who are pregnant should not travel to areas of Brazil with an elevation of under 6,500 feet. Areas above that elevation are believed to be safe because the mosquitoes that spread the virus are generally unable to live at that elevation. If you're considering travel to Brazil, keep reading to understand the risks that Zika may play in your travel plans.

Infections

So far, Brazil has around 100,000 confirmed cases of Zika in 2016. The actual number of infected Brazilians is likely to be higher, as many infected people do not show symptoms of the disease. There have been approximately 1,800 cases of microcephaly in Brazil during the current Zika epidemic.[6]

Traveling to Brazil

Many people have special questions and concerns about travel to Brazil. Some of the top questions include whether travel to Brazil is still allowed, and whether Americans who get sick in Brazil can return to the US Luckily, the answer to both of these questions is yes. The CDC has explained the situation in detail:

Are there travel restrictions to Brazil because of Zika?

No, there are no travel restrictions to Brazil. CDC recommends taking precautions to avoid Zika in Brazil.

If I get sick while I am in Brazil, will I be able to come back to the US?

Yes, you will be able to return to the United States if you are sick. There are no restrictions for travelers entering the United States who may have gotten Zika virus.

CDC has routine steps to detect sick travelers entering the United States, including requirements for ships and airplanes arriving in the United States to report certain illnesses to CDC. State and territorial health departments routinely notify CDC when cases of Zika are detected in the United States. CDC does recommend that if you are too sick to travel, it is best to stay where you are until you are well enough to travel.

Traveling to Brazil if you're expecting

Zika's most important risk factors are for pregnant women and their unborn children. For this reason, it is extremely important to exercise care when traveling to an infected country or region. Since Brazil is the epicenter of the epidemic, it is wise to postpone or cancel travel if you or your loved one is expecting. The CDC recommends that women who are pregnant avoid most travel to Brazil with these guidelines:

Women who are pregnant

Should not travel to any area of Brazil below 6,500 feet. If you must travel to one of these areas, talk to your doctor first and strictly follow steps to prevent mosquito bites during your trip. If your itinerary is limited entirely to areas above 6,500 feet, there is minimal risk of getting Zika from a mosquito.

If you have a partner who lives in or has traveled to Brazil, either use condoms (or other barriers to prevent infection) or do not have sex (vaginal, anal, or oral) during your pregnancy.

Women who are trying to become pregnant

Before you or your partner travel, talk to your doctor about your plans to become pregnant and the risk of Zika virus infection. See CDC guidance for how long you should wait to get pregnant after travel to Brazil. You and your partner should strictly follow steps to prevent mosquito bites.

People who have traveled to Brazil and have a pregnant partner should use condoms or not have sex (vaginal, anal, or oral) during the pregnancy.

Mosquitoes and High Elevation

Most people are not aware that there are certain parts of Brazil (and other countries) where it is very difficult to get Zika from mosquitoes. Although most parts of Brazil are home to the mosquito that carries Zika, there are certain high-elevation locations that do not have a climate suitable for the insect, thus making mosquito-borne transmission of the virus highly unlikely. If you must go to Brazil or another location suffering from Zika outbreaks, consider visiting high-altitude locations instead of low-lying areas. Although the guide below is tailored to Brazil, the same advice should apply to all high-altitude locations. The CDC created a valuable FAQ which answers many questions about the risk of getting Zika at elevations above 6,500 feet, which is excerpted in part below:

What is the risk of getting Zika at high elevations?

The mosquitoes that spread Zika usually do not live at elevations above 6,500 feet (2,000 meters). Travelers who plan to be only in areas above this elevation are at a very low risk of getting Zika from a mosquito. Travelers are still at risk of sexual transmission of Zika.

What if I am flying into an airport at a low elevation in an area with Zika but then immediately driving to a high elevation?

You would still be at risk of getting Zika from a mosquito bite while you were at the low elevation. You should strictly follow steps to prevent mosquito bites while in these areas.

I am going to an area that looks like it is in the high-elevation zone, but your map is not detailed enough for me to see for certain. Is this destination in the risk area?

Talk to your doctor about your risk of Zika in the area where you are traveling. Travelers to destinations that cross or are near an elevation border may consider the destination as an area of lower elevation and follow recommendations for travel to areas with Zika.

What data sources did you use to show that mosquitoes do not usually live above 6,500 feet?

Aedes species mosquitoes, the mosquitoes that carry Zika, live in areas with certain ecological conditions (temperature, rainfall patterns, local plant growth, and human population density). CDC used elevation data to predict areas where the *Aedes* mosquitoes are unlikely to live. Our findings show that *Aedes* mosquitoes are not usually found above 6,500 feet (2,000 meters).

What do you recommend for pregnant women who decide to travel to high elevations in an area with Zika?

The risk of getting Zika from a mosquito at elevations above 6,500 feet (2,000 meters) is minimal. However, traveling through an area of low elevation or stopping even briefly in a low-elevation area on the way to higher elevation increases the risk of getting Zika from a mosquito, and pregnant women should strictly follow steps to prevent mosquito bites while in these areas. Pregnant women traveling to these areas should use condoms or not have sex with partners who may have traveled to lower elevations in an area with Zika. Pregnant women should also be alert to changes in their travel plans that may take them to elevations below 6,500 feet.

Besides Zika, is it safe for pregnant women to travel to high elevations?

The low oxygen levels found at high elevations can cause problems for travelers who are going to elevations above 8,000 feet (2,400 meters). The best way to prevent altitude illness is to ascend slowly and take time to get used to the lower oxygen levels. Pregnant women should avoid strenuous activities at high elevations, and some doctors recommend that pregnant women not spend the night at altitudes above 12,000 feet (3,650 meters). Pregnant women should also consider whether they will have access to medical care at a high-elevation destination.

The situation in Brazil is constantly changing and evolving. Be sure to check out the latest news at cdc.gov/zika, or consult the

US consulate in Brazil to determine the current health situation in the country.

US Embassy Brasilia

SES 801- Avenida das Nacoes, Lote 03

70403–900— Brasilia, DF Brazil

Telephone: 011–55–61–3312–7000

Emergency After-Hours Telephone: 011–55–61–3312–7400

Fax: (61) 3312–7651

BrasiliaACS@state.gov

https://br.usembassy.gov

MEXICO

Overview

Mexico is the most popular destination in the entire world for American tourists. With over twenty million trips made by Americans to Mexico in 2014,[7] Mexico is far and away the most visited foreign destination. While Mexico is an amazing country with fantastic food, beautiful beaches, and a welcoming people, the country has also suffered from the Zika epidemic, making it important to arm yourself with knowledge to protect yourself and your family. Many Mexican cities are located at high elevations over 6,500 feet (2,000 meters). These places are believed to be relatively protected from the mosquitoes that spread Zika, as they cannot generally survive at altitudes that high. For more information on Zika and high altitudes, read the portion on high altitudes in the Brazil section, located just before the Mexico section.

Infections

As of August 15, 2016, Mexico has more than 1,600 confirmed cases of Zika.[8] While this number is much less than hard-hit countries like Brazil and Colombia, it is important to remember that only around 20 percent of people infected with the virus display symptoms, so the real number may be higher. Furthermore, if you are going to Mexico to enjoy the beach, remember that you are likely to be a prime target for mosquitoes, given that most of your body may be uncovered.

Traveling to Mexico

Many people have special questions and concerns about travel to Mexico. Given the popularity of the country as a major tourist destination, understanding how you can protect yourself is extremely important. If you are pregnant, the CDC currently does not recommend you travel to Mexico. The CDC has explained the situation in detail:

What is the current situation?

Local mosquito transmission of Zika virus infection (Zika) has been reported in Mexico. Local mosquito transmission means that mosquitoes in the area are infected with Zika virus and are spreading it to people.

Because Zika virus is primarily spread by mosquitoes, CDC recommends that travelers to Mexico protect themselves from mosquito bites. The mosquitoes that spread Zika usually do not live at elevations above 6,500 feet (2,000 meters) because of environmental conditions. Travelers whose itineraries are limited to areas above this elevation are at minimal risk of getting Zika from a mosquito.

Sexual transmission of Zika virus is also possible, so travelers are encouraged to use condoms (or other barriers to prevent infection) or not have sex. Many people infected with Zika virus do not get sick. Among those who do develop symptoms, sickness is usually mild, with symptoms that last for several days to a week.

Guillain-Barré syndrome (GBS) is a rare disorder that can cause muscle weakness and paralysis for a few weeks to several months. Current CDC research suggests that GBS is strongly associated with Zika; however, only a small proportion of people with recent Zika virus infection get GBS. Most people fully recover from GBS, but some have permanent damage.

What can travelers do to prevent Zika?

There is no vaccine or medicine for Zika. Travelers can protect themselves by preventing mosquito bites:

- Cover exposed skin by wearing long-sleeved shirts and long pants.
- Use EPA-registered insect repellents containing DEET, picaridin, oil of lemon eucalyptus (OLE, also called para-menthane-diol [PMD]), or IR3535. Always use as directed.
  - Pregnant and breastfeeding women can use all EPA-registered insect repellents, including DEET, according to the product label.
  - Most repellents, including DEET, can be used on children older than two months. (OLE should not be used on children younger than three years.)
- Use permethrin-treated clothing and gear (such as boots, pants, socks, and tents). You can buy pre-treated clothing and gear or treat them yourself.
- Stay in places with air conditioning and window and door screens to keep mosquitoes outside.
- Sleep under a mosquito bed net if air conditioned or screened rooms are not available or if sleeping outdoors.

- Mosquito netting can be used to cover babies younger than two months old in carriers, strollers, or cribs to protect them from mosquito bites.

Because Zika can be sexually transmitted, if you have sex (vaginal, anal, or oral) while traveling, you should use condoms.

After travel

Many people infected with Zika virus do not feel sick. If a mosquito bites an infected person while the virus is still in that person's blood, it can spread the virus by biting another person. **Even if they do not feel sick, travelers returning to the United States from Mexico should take steps to prevent mosquito bites for three weeks so that they do not spread Zika to uninfected mosquitoes.**

Travelers returning from Mexico who have a pregnant partner should either use condoms or not have sex for the rest of the pregnancy.

People who have traveled to Mexico should use condoms for at least eight weeks after travel to protect their sex partners. Men who have Zika symptoms or are diagnosed with Zika should use condoms for at least six months after symptoms start; women with symptoms should use condoms for at least eight weeks after symptoms start.

Travelers who are thinking about pregnancy should talk with their health care provider. Men who have traveled to Mexico should wait at least eight weeks after travel before trying to conceive or at least six months after symptoms start if they develop symptoms of Zika. Women who have traveled to Mexico should wait at least eight weeks after travel before trying to get pregnant, or at least eight weeks after symptoms start if they develop symptoms.

If you feel sick and think you may have Zika

- Talk to your doctor if you develop a fever with a rash, joint pain, or red eyes. Tell him or her about your travel.
- Take acetaminophen (paracetamol) to relieve fever and pain. Do not take aspirin, products containing aspirin, or other nonsteroidal anti-inflammatory drugs, such as ibuprofen.
- Get lots of rest and drink plenty of liquids.

If you are pregnant
Talk to a doctor or other health care provider after your trip, **even if you don't feel sick**. Pregnant travelers returning from Mexico or who have had possible sexual exposure should be offered testing for Zika virus infection.

- If you develop a fever with a rash, joint pain, or red eyes, talk to your doctor immediately and tell him or her about your travel or possible sexual exposure.
- If you do not have symptoms, testing should be offered if you see a health care provider up to twelve weeks after you return from travel or your last possible sexual exposure.

Zika virus in pregnancy
A pregnant woman can pass Zika virus to her fetus. Infection during pregnancy can cause serious birth defects. CDC recommends special precautions for the following groups:

- Women who are pregnant:
  - Should not travel to any area of Mexico below 6,500 feet (see map).

- If you must travel to one of these areas, talk to your doctor first and strictly follow steps to prevent mosquito bites during your trip. If your itinerary is limited **entirely** to areas above 6,500 feet, there is minimal risk of getting Zika from a mosquito.
- If you have a partner who lives in or has traveled to Mexico, either use condoms (or other barriers to prevent infection) or do not have sex (vaginal, anal, or oral) during your pregnancy.
- Women who are trying to become pregnant:
  - Before you or your partner travel, talk to your doctor about your plans to become pregnant and the risk of Zika virus infection.
  - See CDC guidance for how long you should wait to get pregnant after travel to Mexico.
  - You and your partner should strictly follow steps to prevent mosquito bites.

If you are traveling in Mexico and need assistance, don't hesitate to contact the US Embassy. Remember, the situation is always changing and asking for updated information on Zika is always a smart choice. You can also find out more at www.cdc.gov/zika

Embassy of the United States in Mexico City
Paseo de la Reforma 305
Colonia Cuauhtemoc
06500 Mexico, D.F.

Telephones:
From Mexico:
Tel : (01–55) 5080–2000
Fax: (01–55) 5080–2005

From the US:
Tel: 011–52–55–5080–2000
Fax: 011–52–55–5080–2005
acsmexicocity@state.gov
https://mx.usembassy.gov

PUERTO RICO

Overview

Puerto Rico is a US territory located in the Caribbean. With its close proximity to countries with high infection rates, and a climate in which mosquitoes thrive, it is a rich territory for the spread of the Zika virus. Several bungled attempts to cull the mosquito population have contributed to the robust spread of Zika in the territory. Furthermore, a looming debt crisis has hampered government efforts to take decisive action.

Infections

As of August 2016, there are currently more than 10,000 confirmed cases in Puerto Rico. The actual number of Zika cases is believed to be substantially higher because around 80 percent of people infected with Zika report no symptoms. Most of these people probably don't even know they are infected. The Surgeon General estimated that one-fourth of people in Puerto Rico will be infected with Zika by the end of 2016.[9] Given that Puerto Rico has a population of approximately 3.5 million, around 875,000 people could be at risk by the end of 2016.

Health Emergency

On August 12, 2016, a health emergency was declared in Puerto Rico. Secretary of Health and Human Services Sylvia Mathews Burwell vowed to strenuously fight the virus, declaring, "This

Administration is committed to meeting the Zika outbreak in Puerto Rico with the necessary urgency." She went on to note the importance of fighting Zika, outlining the risks and challenges that the virus poses:

"As the first virus that can be transmitted by mosquitoes known to cause severe birth defects, we are working closely with Puerto Rican officials to pursue solutions to fight the virus in Puerto Rico with a focus on protecting pregnant women and continuing our efforts with jurisdictions throughout the United States to address this public health threat."

Crucially, she said that the declaration would make it easier for the funds to flow to Puerto Rico to help address the Zika epidemic.

"This emergency declaration allows us to provide additional support to the Puerto Rican government and reminds us of the importance of pregnant women, women of childbearing age, and their partners taking additional steps to protect themselves and their families from Zika."

Puerto Rico is the center of the Zika epidemic in the United States, so it is crucial that the US and Puerto Rican governments work together to solve this crisis. This order is a step in the right direction and signals that both governments are taking the problem seriously.

Traveling to Puerto Rico if you're expecting

Zika virus in pregnancy
Zika's most important risk factors are for pregnant women and their unborn children. For this reason, it is extremely important to exercise care when traveling to an infected country or region. Since Puerto Rico has a very high Zika infection rate, it is wise to

postpone or cancel travel if you or your loved one is expecting. The CDC recommends that women who are pregnant avoid most travel to Puerto Rico:

A pregnant woman can pass Zika virus to her fetus. Infection during pregnancy can cause serious birth defects. CDC recommends special precautions for the following groups:

Women who are pregnant

Should not travel to Puerto Rico. If you must travel, talk to your doctor first and strictly follow steps to prevent mosquito bites during your trip. If you have a partner who lives in or has traveled to Puerto Rico, either use condoms (or other barriers to prevent infection) or do not have sex (vaginal, anal, or oral) during your pregnancy.

Women who are trying to become pregnant

Before you or your partner travel, talk to your doctor about your plans to become pregnant and the risk of Zika virus infection. See CDC guidance for how long you should wait to get pregnant after travel to Puerto Rico.

You and your partner should strictly follow steps to prevent mosquito bites.

People who have traveled to Puerto Rico and have a pregnant partner should use condoms or not have sex (vaginal, anal, or oral) during the pregnancy.

After returning from Puerto Rico

If you do travel to Puerto Rico, be sure to take appropriate precautions to protect you, your family, and your community after you return. The CDC recommends:

Many people infected with Zika virus do not feel sick. If a mosquito bites an infected person while the virus is still in that person's blood, it can spread the virus by biting another person. **Even if they do not feel sick, travelers returning to the United States from Puerto Rico should take steps to prevent mosquito bites for three weeks so that they do not spread Zika to uninfected mosquitoes.**

Travelers returning from Puerto Rico who have a pregnant partner should either use condoms or not have sex for the rest of the pregnancy.

People who have traveled to Puerto Rico should use condoms for at least 8 weeks after travel to protect their sex partners. Men who have Zika symptoms or are diagnosed with Zika should use condoms for at least 6 months after symptoms start; women with symptoms should use condoms for at least eight weeks after symptoms start.

Travelers who are thinking about pregnancy should talk with their health care provider. Men who have traveled to Puerto Rico should wait at least eight weeks after travel before trying to conceive or at least six months after symptoms start if they develop symptoms of Zika. Women who have traveled to Puerto Rico should wait at least eight weeks after travel before trying to get pregnant, or at least eight weeks after symptoms start if they develop symptoms.

Regardless of why you're traveling to Puerto Rico, use caution and avoid mosquito bites. Also be sure to practice safe sexual practices—covered in a later chapter—to prevent the sexual spread of the virus. Updated information on the situation in Puerto Rico can be found at cdc.gov/zika.

Puerto Rico Department of Health
Centro Médico Norte
Calle Periferial Interior,
Bo. Monacillos Rio Piedras, PR

(787) 765–2929
contactus@salud.pr.gov
http://www.salud.gov.pr

Note: While Puerto Rico is a US territory, government agencies generally conduct business in Spanish. You may be not be able to easily reach someone who speaks English.

FLORIDA

Overview

Miami is one of America's great cities, with beautiful beaches and friendly people, so the news that it was the first location in the continental US with local Zika transmission was unnerving for many Americans. It wasn't just a seemingly distant threat, restricted to foreign countries or American territories apart from the mainland. As of June 15, 2016, it's here now. The CDC has released information regarding travel to the Wynwood and Miami Beach areas of Miami, covered after the infections section below.

Infections

As of August 2016, Florida has suffered nearly 500 confirmed travel-related cases of Zika. Confirmed locally transmitted cases of Zika are at thirty-six and rising. For the most recent figures, contact the Florida Department of Health, or visit the CDC's Zika website at cdc.gov/zika.

Travel warning

The Florida Department of Health has identified two areas of Miami-Dade County where Zika is being spread by mosquitoes. In addition to the previously identified area in the Wynwood neighborhood, there is now mosquito-borne spread of Zika virus in a section of Miami Beach.

This guidance is for people who live in or traveled to the identified area of Miami Beach any time after July 14. This guidance also still applies for those who live in or traveled to the previously identified Wynwood area any time after June 15. These timeframes are based on the earliest time symptoms can start and the maximum two-week incubation period for Zika virus.

Pregnant women and their partners

- Pregnant women should not travel to these areas.
- Pregnant women and their partners living in or traveling to these areas should follow steps to prevent mosquito bites.
- Women and men who live in or traveled to these areas and who have a pregnant sex partner should use condoms or other barriers to prevent infection every time they have sex, or not have sex during the pregnancy.
- Pregnant women and their partners who are concerned about being exposed to Zika may want to consider postponing nonessential travel to all parts of Miami-Dade County.
- All pregnant women in the United States should be assessed for possible Zika virus exposure during each prenatal care visit.
- Pregnant women who live in or frequently travel to these areas should be tested in the first and second trimesters of pregnancy.
- Pregnant women with possible Zika exposure and signs or symptoms of Zika should be tested for Zika.

- Pregnant women who traveled to or had unprotected sex with a partner that traveled to or lives in these areas should talk to their healthcare provider and should be tested for Zika.

Couples thinking about getting pregnant

- Women with Zika should wait at least eight weeks and men with Zika should wait at least six months after symptoms began to try to get pregnant.
- Women and men who live in or frequently travel to these areas should talk to their healthcare provider.
- Women and men who traveled to these areas should wait at least eight weeks before trying to get pregnant.

For questions on mosquito control in Florida

Florida health officials can answer specific questions on their mosquito control program. Aerial treatment of areas with products that rapidly reduce both young and adult mosquitoes can help to limit the number of mosquitoes that carry the Zika virus. Repeated aerial applications of insecticide has reduced mosquito populations as a part of an integrated vector management program.

If you have questions about Zika in Florida, be sure to contact the Florida Department of Health.

Florida Department of Health
Phone: 850–245–4444
Email: health@flhealth.gov
Mailing Address
Florida Department of Health
4052 Bald Cypress Way
Tallahassee, FL 32399

VENEZUELA

Safety in a precarious time

Venezuela, situated just north of Brazil, has also been hit hard by the Zika virus. However, travelers to this beautiful country have more than just Zika to worry about. As of 2016 the country is in the midst of a crushing economic and political crisis, making travel dangerous in more ways than one. The same Zika risks that exist in Brazil are also extant in Venezuela, and you should consult the Brazil section for Zika-specific warnings and tips. However, given the economic crisis, the healthcare system cannot be depended on. Reuters reported that local Venezuelan women are undergoing sterilization rather than risk unplanned pregnancies, because the country has run out of birth control. Medical shortages are said to run at 85 percent, signaling a dramatic lack of available medical care.[10] If you get sick in Venezuela, leaving the country might be key to protecting your health.

While any travelers to Venezuela should of course take all precautions to avoid the Zika virus, they should also be aware of these special risks identified by the Bureau of Consular Affairs, US State Department:

The Department of State warns US citizens that violent crime in Venezuela is pervasive, both in the capital Caracas and throughout the country. Security restrictions on US government personnel may restrict the services the Embassy can provide. All US direct-hire personnel and their families assigned to the US Embassy in Caracas are subject to an embassy movement policy which limits their travel abilities within Caracas and in other parts of the country for their safety and well-being. Country-wide shortages of food, water, medicine, electricity, and other basic goods have led to violence and looting. This replaces the Travel Warning issued on September 18, 2015.

Venezuela has one of the world's highest crime rates and, according to the non-governmental organization Venezuelan Violence Observatory, has the second highest homicide rate. Violent crime—including murder, armed robbery, kidnapping, and carjacking—is endemic throughout the country. Drug traffickers and illegal armed groups are active in the Colombian border states of Zulia, Tachira, and Apure.

Armed robberies and street crime take place throughout Caracas and other cities, including in areas generally presumed safe and frequented by tourists. Heavily armed criminals are known to use grenades and assault rifles to commit crimes at banks, shopping malls, public transportation stations, and universities. Criminals may take advantage of power outages to target victims when lights and security alarms are nonfunctional.

Political rallies and demonstrations can occur with little notice, and are expected to occur with greater frequency in the coming months in Caracas and other regions throughout the country. Long lines to purchase basic goods are a common occurrence throughout the country and there have been reports of unrest and violence while customers wait, sometimes resulting in looted stores and blocked streets. These incidents elicit a strong police and security force response that can include the use of violence against the participants; several deaths have been reported during such protests.

Although Venezuela is a signatory to the Vienna Convention on Consular Relations, the Venezuelan government sometimes fails to notify the US Embassy when US citizens are arrested, and/ or delays or denies consular access to arrestees. In cases where individuals hold dual citizenship, we are not guaranteed consular access to the detained individuals. Regardless, the US Embassy makes it a priority to request access to US citizens, but US citizens cannot assume a consular officer will visit them within 24–72 hours of an arrest.

For further information on preventing Zika infection while in Venezuela, consult the sections on Brazil Travel and Prevention. For the latest on Venezuela's special political and economic risks, visit the State Department at travel.state.gov or contact the US Embassy.

US Embassy Caracas
Calle F con Calle Suapure,
Urb. Colinas de Valle Arriba,
Caracas, Venezuela 1080
Telephone: +(58) (212) 975–6411
Emergency After-Hours Telephone: +(58) (212) 907–8400
Fax: +(58) (212) 907–8199
ACSVenezuela@state.gov

WHAT TO DO AFTER TRAVELING TO A LOCATION WITH ZIKA

It is crucial to protect yourself and your family after travel to a location with Zika. For detailed CDC advice on how to protect yourself and your loved ones after potential exposure to Zika, be sure to read the "After Returning from Puerto Rico" section of this chapter. It contains valuable CDC advice that should be applicable even if you have traveled to another country or territory with Zika.

As mentioned in the above CDC advice, it is crucial that you avoid potentially infecting others with the virus, particularly if your partner is pregnant. If your partner is expecting and you have reason to believe you may be infected with Zika, be sure to abstain from sexual activity or use condoms until the child is delivered. Doing otherwise may expose the baby to the risk of contracting Zika and developing microcephaly.

WHAT TO DO IF YOU LIVE SOMEWHERE WITH ZIKA

The CDC has created guidelines for women living in Wynwood, Miami—the only area of the continental US hit by the local transmission of Zika. These guidelines are likely to apply to anywhere struck by the virus and are adapted here:

Pregnant women and their partners

- Pregnant women should not travel to this area.
- Pregnant women and their partners living in or traveling to this area should follow steps to prevent mosquito bites.
- Women and men who live in or traveled to this area and who have a pregnant sex partner should use condoms or other barriers to prevent infection every time they have sex or not have sex during the pregnancy.
- All pregnant women in the United States should be assessed for possible Zika virus exposure during each prenatal care visit.
- Pregnant women who **live in** or **frequently travel** to this area should be tested in the first and second trimesters of pregnancy.
- Pregnant women with possible Zika exposure and signs or symptoms of Zika should be tested for Zika.

- Pregnant women who traveled to or had unprotected sex with a partner who traveled to or lives in this area should talk to their healthcare provider and should be tested for Zika.

Couples thinking about getting pregnant

- Women with Zika should wait at least eight weeks and men with Zika should wait at least six months after symptoms began to try to get pregnant.
- Women and men who live in or frequently travel to this area should talk to their healthcare provider.
- Women and men who traveled to this area should wait at least eight weeks before trying to get pregnant.

WHAT ARE OTHER COUNTRIES DOING TO HELP?

Governments around the world have responded to the Zika epidemic, but not all of them have the same resources to deal with the problem. Some of the hardest-hit countries are developing or middle-income countries with healthcare systems that are not as advanced as they could be. Furthermore, many of these countries are close to the equator, meaning that the mosquitoes that spread Zika can survive year-round.

The epidemic has also exacerbated geopolitical tensions. Colombia and Venezuela, long regional rivals, have seen their relationship continue to be strained by the crisis. Venezuela has refused to coordinate medical care or even talk to Colombia about the issue. Colombia has also accused Venezuela of deliberately underreporting Zika cases.[11] Venezuela, which is the in midst of a major political and economic crisis, lacks adequate supplies of medicine, birth control, and even food.

Zika is spread over a large region, making elimination of the mosquitoes that carry the virus nearly impossible. The chaotic situation in Venezuela and the differing responses by governments around the region means that even if certain countries eradicate Zika within their borders—an already nearly impossible task— it will simply begin to spread again from surrounding areas. In short, as long as there is no vaccine, mitigation is the only true option for governments now. Cuba, which has a longstanding and extensive fumigation apparatus, has been particularly successful in this regard, although given its location in the Caribbean, even those extensive measures have been unable to completely eliminate the threat.

Brazil, hardest hit by the crisis, has massively mobilized its citizens to fight against the virus. The government has organized over 500,000 people, including members of the armed forces, government employees, and citizen volunteers.[12] Still, despite these efforts, Brazil has thus far been unable to stop the spread of the virus.

In the United States, work on a vaccine has continued, and there are promising developments. On August 4, 2016, researchers working at the Walter Reed Army Institute of Research and Harvard's Beth Israel Hospital reported a breakthrough which some believe will lead to the first safe and effective Zika vaccine for humans.[13] One reason that this research seems so promising is that all three of the vaccine test candidates were found safe and effective in monkeys. Earlier results had suggested effectiveness in mice, but monkeys are a much closer match to humans. Although all three have shown progress, only the most promising of the three potential vaccines under development, known as the

ZPIV vaccine, will progress to human trials that should start in October of 2016.

3

Transcription

OVERVIEW

If you don't have Zika, the only way to get it is from someone who does. Sure, getting Zika from a mosquito might be indirect, but nevertheless, that mosquito got the virus from another human. Aside from mosquito-borne transmission, Zika has been found in blood, saliva, vaginal and seminal fluid, amniotic fluid in the womb, and breast milk. Thus the virus has multiple ways of spreading.

Zika is currently known to spread through mosquito bites, "vertical transmission" from a pregnant mother to her unborn child, sexual intercourse, general exposure, or blood transfusions. Despite Zika being present in some breast milk, there are still no confirmed transmissions through breast milk, and the CDC encourages women to continue to breastfeed their babies.

Initial infections of Zika are primarily caused by mosquito bites. This is the most common way the virus spreads, and why it has reached epidemic levels in certain South American countries. Zika that has infected a pregnant woman can also spread to her unborn child. This method of transmission is extremely rare for a mosquito-borne virus, and one of the things that makes Zika unique. Furthermore, Zika can be spread from one infected person to another through sexual intercourse. Although it was initially believed to be spread from exclusively from men to their sexual partners, it is now confirmed that women can pass on

Zika as well. Since Zika is present in the blood of those infected with the virus, blood transfusions with Zika-tainted blood are yet another way to spread the virus.

MOSQUITOES

Mosquitoes are the most common way Zika is spread, and the method of spreading the disease that is most associated with the disease in the popular consciousness.

The CDC has identified and describes two types of mosquitoes, the *Aedes aegypti* (yellow fever mosquito), and the *Aedes albopictus* (Asian tiger mosquito), as the primary spreaders of the Zika virus.

Aedes aegypti

- These mosquitoes live in tropical, subtropical, and in some temperate climates.
- They are the main type of mosquito that spreads Zika, dengue, chikungunya, and other viruses.
- Because *Aedes aegypti* mosquitoes live near and prefer to feed on people, they are more likely to spread these viruses than other types of mosquitoes.

Aedes albopictus

- These mosquitoes live tropical, subtropical, and temperate climates, but can live in a broader temperature range and at cooler temperatures than *Aedes aegypti*.
- Because these mosquitoes feed on animals as well as people, they are less likely to spread viruses like Zika, dengue, chikungunya, and other viruses.

About outbreaks spread by mosquitoes

- Local mosquito-borne Zika virus transmission has been reported in the continental United States.
- Many areas in the United States have the type of mosquitoes that can become infected with and spread Zika, chikungunya, and dengue viruses.
- Recent outbreaks in the continental United States of chikungunya and dengue, which are spread by the same type of mosquito, have been relatively small and limited to a small area.
- Areas with past outbreaks of chikungunya and dengue are considered at higher risk for Zika. These include US territories like Puerto Rico, the US Virgin Islands, and Guam. Local outbreaks have also been reported in parts of Hawaii, Florida, and Texas.
- *Aedes aegypti* or *Aedes albopictus* mosquitoes can cause an outbreak, if all of the following happens:
  - People get infected with a virus (like Zika, dengue, or chikungunya).
  - An *Aedes aegypti* or *Aedes albopictus* mosquito bites an infected person during the first week of infection, when the virus can be found in the person's blood.
  - The infected mosquito lives long enough for the virus to multiply and for the mosquito to bite another person.
  - The cycle continues multiple times to start an outbreak.

VERTICAL TRANSMISSION (MOTHER TO CHILD)

The strangest and most important way Zika is transmitted is from a pregnant mother to her unborn child. Studies suggest that Zika can breach the placental barrier, which can often protect the still-developing child from threats extant in the mother's blood. Zika's case is particularly strange because many mosquito-borne viruses are not able to breach the placental barrier.

Zika transmission to an unborn child is the most well-known, and most dangerous, risk created by Zika. If the unborn child is infected, they are at risk of suffering from microcephaly, which causes smaller-than-average head size and retards brain development.

Vertical transmission is a serious issue, and the CDC has released this information on the issue:

- A pregnant woman can pass Zika virus to her fetus during pregnancy. Zika is a cause of microcephaly and other severe fetal brain defects. [The CDC is] studying the full range of other potential health problems that Zika virus infection during pregnancy may cause.
- A pregnant woman already infected with Zika virus can pass the virus to her fetus during the pregnancy or around the time of birth.
- To date, there are no reports of infants getting Zika virus through breastfeeding. Because of the benefits of breastfeeding, mothers are encouraged to breastfeed even in areas where Zika virus is found.

SEXUAL INTERCOURSE

Although it was once believed that only men could pass Zika to their partners through sexual intercourse, recent evidence suggests that women infected with the virus can also pass it on to their sexual partners. Margaret Chan, director of the

World Health Organization (WHO), said,[14] "Of course, we also have learnt from the latest evidence it's not just infected men who can pass the disease to their sex partners. There was a case of a lady passing the disease to a man, so it can go both directions." Zika can spread both through vaginal and anal sexual intercourse, meaning that both genders and people of all sexual orientations are potentially vulnerable to the sexual spread of the virus.

There is limited but growing evidence that the sexual transmission of Zika may become a large problem and a key way the virus spreads. One man in France had a viral load of Zika in his semen "roughly 100,000 times that of his blood or urine more than two weeks after symptom onset."[15] This suggests that Zika, at least in some cases, has a significant susceptibility to be spread through sexual contact. Moreover, according to the CDC, "Zika can remain in semen longer than in other body fluids, including vaginal fluids, urine, and blood." This suggests that infected men and their partners need to pay particular care during sexual activity, or abstain from it altogether. Mounting evidence suggests that the sexual transmission of Zika could become a serious problem. One man in Italy was found to have Zika in his semen a full six months after contracting the virus—twice as long as any previous case. This has led to some to speculate that the virus can replicate itself within the male genital tract.[16]

The CDC has issued advice regarding sexual activity and Zika:

- Zika can be passed through sex from a person who has Zika to his or her partners. Zika can be passed through sex, even if the infected person does not have symptoms at the time.

- It can be passed from a person with Zika before their symptoms start, while they have symptoms, and after their symptoms end.
- Though not well documented, the virus may also be passed by a person who carries the virus but never develops symptoms.
- Studies are under way to find out how long Zika stays in the semen and vaginal fluids of people who have Zika, and how long it can be passed to sex partners. We know that Zika can remain in semen longer than in other body fluids, including vaginal fluids, urine, and blood.

EXPOSURE

Exposure to Zika patients or family members may facilitate the spread of the virus, particularly if there is contact with blood or other bodily fluids. Merely being around someone with Zika is unlikely to give you the virus, although a mosquito that bites the infected person before biting you may give you the virus.

However, even without such exposure, there is limited evidence that other still-unknown forms of transmission may be possible. A strange case that attracted widespread media attention involved a since-deceased elderly man in Utah who contracted Zika while traveling to an infected country. A person living in the same household, identified by some media sources as the man's son, also contracted the disease. This was highly unusual as there was no contact between the residents that, in a typical case, would allow transmission of the virus. Furthermore, Utah is not home to the type of mosquitoes that spread Zika. The viral load in the elderly man was found to be more than 100,000 times greater than those seen in other infected people. The CDC released this media statement in regards to that strange case:

CDC is assisting in the investigation of a case of Zika in a Utah resident who is a family contact of the elderly Utah resident who died in late June. The deceased patient had traveled to an area with Zika and lab tests showed he had uniquely high amounts of virus—more than 100,000 times higher than seen in other samples of infected people—in his blood. Laboratories in Utah and at the Centers for Disease Control and Prevention (CDC) reported evidence of Zika infection in both Utah residents.

State and local public health disease control specialists, along with CDC, are investigating how the second resident became infected. The investigation includes additional interviews with and laboratory testing of family members and healthcare workers who may have had contact with the person who died and trapping mosquitoes and assessing the risk of local spread by mosquitoes.

It is not just average people living in afflicted areas who can find themselves at risk. Those who treat or study Zika also face the possibility of infection. As the CDC has noted, there have been multiple cases of laboratory transmission of Zika.

- Prior to the current outbreak, there were four reports of laboratory-acquired Zika virus infections, although the route of transmission was not clearly established in all cases.
- As of June 15, 2016, there has been one reported case of laboratory-acquired Zika virus disease in the United States.

BLOOD TRANSFUSIONS

There is nothing scarier than having to second-guess whether the blood that is needed to keep patients safe and save lives is safe to use. Yet this is the dilemma facing public health professionals as Zika spreads. The CDC has issued this information concerning Zika and the potential risks posed by blood transfusions:

- Zika virus currently poses a low risk to the blood supply in the continental US, but this could change depending on how many people become infected with the virus.
- There is a strong possibility that Zika virus can be spread through blood transfusions.
  - Because most people infected with the Zika virus don't show any symptoms, blood donors may not know they have been infected.
  - There have been cases of Zika transmission through blood transfusion in Brazil. During the previous French Polynesian Zika virus outbreak, 2.8 percent of blood donors tested positive for Zika, and in previous outbreaks, the virus has been found in blood donors.
- In areas of active transmission, FDA recommends that blood either be screened by laboratory testing, subjected to pathogen reduction technology (PRT), or outsourced from other areas.

It might sound implausible for the CDC to suggest that blood be outsourced from other areas, but remember, Zika is a regional virus. Although it is infecting Americans, there are large areas of the United States where it is unlikely to become endemic. Zika is unlikely to spread widely in cold climates, particularly during the winter. Thus, the US, Canada, and Northern Europe should be able to maintain regions with a comparatively safe blood-donation population, even if the virus continues to infect more people.

Regrettably, the CDC says, "Blood donor screening on the basis of a questionnaire, without a laboratory test, is insufficient for identifying Zika-infected donors in areas with active mosquito-borne transmission of Zika virus due to the high rate of asymptomatic infection." Thus, other more stringent methods of protecting the blood supply and preventing contamination are necessary.

BREAST MILK

Although the Zika virus has been found in breast milk, the CDC has encouraged women to continue breastfeeding, even in areas with the virus. They note, "To date, there are no reports of infants getting Zika virus through breastfeeding. Because of the benefits of breastfeeding, mothers are encouraged to breastfeed even in areas where Zika virus is found." Current medical knowledge is always changing and advancing, so if you are uncertain whether to breastfeed your baby, be sure to talk to a medical professional or visit the CDC's Zika website at cdc.gov/zika.

4

Prevention

MOSQUITO PROTECTION

The old saying "prevention is the best medicine" certainly applies to Zika. Because there is no cure, preventing getting infected with the virus is your first and most important line of defense. The best way to stay safe is to arm yourself with knowledge, then follow CDC-recommended best practices. While the virus can be spread through sexual activity or blood transfusions, most people get it from mosquitoes. The CDC has multiple recommendations, including using EPA-registered insect repellents as a first line of defense.

What are CDC recommendations for preventing Zika using mosquito repellent?

CDC recommends using EPA-registered insect repellents to prevent mosquito bites. EPA-registered repellents have been tested to make sure that they are both safe and effective.

Pregnant and breastfeeding women can use all EPA-registered insect repellents, including DEET. Most repellents, including DEET, can also be used on children older than two months. (However, OLE should not be used on children younger than three years.)

Which brand of insect repellent should I use? What ingredients should I look for on the label?

CDC doesn't recommend specific repellent brands. Be sure to use EPA-registered repellent containing one of the following ingredients: DEET, picaridin, oil of lemon eucalyptus (OLE, also called PMD), or IR3535. Higher percentages of active ingredient provide longer time periods of protection; for example, CDC recommends using products with at least 20–50 percent DEET.

Note that oil of lemon eucalyptus (OLE) is an EPA-registered ingredient, but "pure" oil of lemon eucalyptus (essential oil not formulated as a repellent) is not recommended. It has not undergone testing for safety and efficacy and is not registered with EPA as an insect repellent.

How effective are natural mosquito repellents?

Insect repellents that are not registered with the EPA, including some natural repellents, perfumes, or essential oils, have not been proven effective. Do not use insect repellents that aren't EPA-registered. There are many products out there; choosing an EPA-registered repellent ensures the EPA has evaluated the product for effectiveness.

Are there any specific kinds of clothes I should bring with me?

If possible, wear long-sleeved shirts and long pants to prevent mosquito bites. You can also use permethrin-treated clothing and gear. You can buy pre-treated clothing and gear or treat them yourself.

ZIKA AND CHILDREN

When traveling with children, take the same precautions with them as you would yourself. Although we know that the effects of Zika can be serious in unborn children, we do not yet know if babies or small children that contract Zika after being born will suffer long-term damage. Because of the uncertainty surrounding the situation, it is best that you take careful precautions to protect your children from the virus. Avoid all nonessential travel to Zika-prone areas, and if you live in one, use extra care. The CDC has recommended several steps for protecting small children from mosquitoes:

- Do not use insect repellents on babies younger than two months old.
- Do not use products containing OLE or PMD on children younger than three years old.
- Children should not touch repellent. Adults should apply it to their hands and gently spread it over the child's exposed skin.
- Do not apply repellent to children's hands because they tend to put their hands in their mouths.
- Keep repellent out of the reach of children.

For babies under two months old, protect them by draping mosquito netting over their carrier or car seat. Netting should have an elastic edge for a tight fit.

TRAVEL MEASURES

Hot Climates

If you're traveling to a country or location with Zika, you're almost certainly going to be feeling the heat. That's because the mosquitoes that spread Zika thrive in hot climates and simply can't survive in the cold. Although avoiding Zika will be a top priority, common-sense measures to stay healthy are a vital part of your travel plans. These CDC recommendations apply to anyone traveling to a hot climate:

Traveling in hot climates can make you sick, especially if you are not accustomed to the heat. People at highest risk are the elderly, young children, and people with chronic illnesses, but even young and healthy people can get sick from heat if they participate in strenuous physical activities during hot weather.

When you are not in an air-conditioned building, take these steps to prevent heat-related illnesses, injuries, and deaths when traveling in hot climates:

- Drink plenty of fluids.
- Wear loose, lightweight, light-colored clothing and sunscreen.
- Try to schedule outdoor activities during cooler parts of the day.
- Rest often, and try to stay in the shade when outdoors.
- If you will be doing strenuous activities in the heat, try to get adjusted before you leave by exercising one hour per day in the heat.

Overheating can result in heat exhaustion or heatstroke. Symptoms include excessive thirst, profuse sweating, headache, dizziness or confusion, and nausea. If you or anyone you are traveling with develops these symptoms, get out of the sun and try to cool off by fanning or getting in the water. Heatstroke is a life-threatening medical emergency; get medical attention if symptoms persist.

GETTING HEALTHCARE ABROAD

Getting a virus in a foreign country isn't fun, but if you think you have contracted Zika and you can't find a way back home, you may need to get care locally. Quality of care will vary widely depending on your location, but the CDC has general guidelines for people in foreign countries who need to get medical care:

Travelers may get sick or injured without warning while traveling, and you should plan in advance how to get care when you're overseas. This applies to all travelers but is especially important for senior citizens, pregnant women, people with preexisting conditions, or people who will be in a foreign country for a long time.

Find a doctor

The US Embassy in your destination country (www.usembassy. gov) can help you locate medical services and will notify your family and friends in the event of an emergency. When selecting a doctor, make sure that he or she can speak your language. The following resources provide lists of doctors and clinics that can care for travelers:

- The International Association for Medical Assistance to Travelers (www.iamat.org; membership required, but it is free)
- Joint Commission International (www.jointcommissioninternational.org)
- The International Society of Travel Medicine (www.istm.org)
- Travel Health Online (www.tripprep.com; gets information from various sources so quality is not guaranteed)

Prepare in advance

Nobody wants to get sick while on a trip, but you can do some simple things to make sure you're prepared, just in case:

- Consider whether you might need travel health or evacuation insurance.
- Register with the US Embassy in your destination country at https://step.state.gov/step/.

- Bring any medicines you may need (pack extra, in case of delays) from the United States. Medicines in other countries may be counterfeit.
- Carry a card that identifies, in the local language, your blood type, any chronic illnesses you have, any medicines you are taking, and any allergies you have.
- Wear a MedicAlert bracelet if you have serious medical conditions.

FOOD SAFETY

If you're traveling somewhere where Zika is a problem, then food might be too. Many of the locations that are experiencing Zika outbreaks are in developing countries. While Zika will be a key worry, you'll also have to be careful what you eat. Local germs and bacteria can give you a wide variety of illnesses, including traveler's diarrhea, sometimes known as Montezuma's revenge. Read these CDC guidelines carefully to help yourself avoid some common developing-world food pitfalls:

Contaminated food or drinks can cause travelers' diarrhea and other diseases. Travelers to developing countries are especially at risk. Reduce your risk by sticking to safe eating and drinking habits.

Food

Usually Safe

Hot food

High heat kills the germs that cause travelers' diarrhea, so food that is cooked thoroughly is usually safe as long as it is served steaming hot. Be careful of food that is cooked and allowed to sit at warm or room temperatures, such as on a buffet. It could become contaminated again.

Dry or packaged food

Most germs require moisture to grow, so food that is dry, such as bread or potato chips, is usually safe. Additionally, food from factory-sealed containers, such as canned tuna or packaged crackers, is safe as long as it was not opened and handled by another person.

Can Be Risky

Raw food

Raw food should generally be avoided. Raw fruits or vegetables may be safe if you can peel them yourself or wash them in safe (bottled or disinfected) water. Steer clear of platters of cut-up fruit or vegetables. (Did you see the hands that cut them? Can you be sure those hands were clean?) Salads are especially problematic because shredded or finely cut vegetables offer a lot of surface area for germs to grow on. Also avoid fresh salsas or other condiments made from raw fruits or vegetables. Raw meat or seafood may contain germs; this includes raw meat that is "cooked" with citrus juice, vinegar, or other acidic liquid (such as ceviche, a dish of raw seafood marinated in citrus juice).

Street food

Street vendors in developing countries may not be held to the same hygiene standards as restaurants (which may be low to begin with), so eat food from street vendors with caution. If you choose to eat street food, apply the same rules as to other food; for example, if you watch something come straight off the grill (cooked and steaming hot), it's more likely to be safe.

Bushmeat

Bushmeat refers to local wild game, generally animals not typically eaten in the United States, such as bats, monkeys, or rodents. Bushmeat can be a source of animal-origin diseases, such as Ebola or SARS, and is best avoided.

Drinks

Usually Safe

Bottled or canned drinks
Drinks from factory-sealed bottles or cans are safe; however, dishonest vendors in some countries may sell tap water in bottles that are "sealed" with a drop of glue to mimic the factory seal. Carbonated drinks, such as sodas or sparkling water, are safest since the bubbles indicate that the bottle was sealed at the factory. If drinking directly from a can, wipe off the lip of the can before your mouth comes into contact with it.

Hot drinks
Hot coffee or tea should be safe if it is served steaming hot. It's okay to let it cool before you drink it, but be wary of coffee or tea that is served only warm or at room temperature. Be careful about adding things that may be contaminated (cream, lemon) to your hot drinks (sugar should be fine; see "Dry food" above).

Milk
Pasteurized milk from a sealed bottle should be okay, but watch out for milk in open containers (such as pitchers) that may have been sitting at room temperature. This includes the cream you put in your coffee or tea. People who are pregnant or have weakened immune systems should stay away from unpasteurized milk or other dairy products (cheese, yogurt).

Alcohol

The alcohol content of most liquors is sufficient to kill germs; however, stick to the guidelines above when choosing mixers and avoid drinks "on the rocks" (see "Ice" below). The alcohol content of beer and wine is probably not high enough to kill germs, but if it came from a sealed bottle or can, it should be okay.

Can Be Risky

Tap water

In most developing countries, tap water should probably not be drunk, even in cities. This includes swallowing water when showering or brushing your teeth. In some areas, it may be advisable to brush your teeth with bottled water. Tap water can be disinfected by boiling, filtering, or chemically treating it, for example with chlorine.

Fountain drinks

Sodas from a fountain are made by carbonating water and mixing it with flavored syrup. Since the water most likely came from the tap, these sodas are best avoided. Similarly, juice from a fountain is most likely juice concentrate mixed with tap water and should be avoided.

Ice

Avoid ice in developing countries; it was likely made with tap water.

Freshly squeezed juice

If you washed the fruit in safe water and squeezed the juice yourself, drink up. Juice that was squeezed by unknown hands may be risky. The same goes for ice pops and other treats that are made from freshly squeezed juice.

CRUISE SHIPS

Cruises can be an amazing experience, but many of the most popular cruise destinations, like Caribbean islands and Central American countries, are also hit hard by the Zika virus. With that in mind, these CDC guidelines can help protect you and your family if you are going on a cruise:

For many people, a cruise is an ideal way to relax and see the world. You are surrounded by the gorgeous blue of the ocean, get waited on hand and foot, have activities and events planned for you, and are provided with a seemingly limitless supply of food and drinks—all while having the opportunity to visit multiple countries and destinations.

Although cruising has many obvious pleasures, potential health hazards are also a risk with cruise ship travel. Staying informed and preparing for these potential hazards can help you stay healthy and get the most out of your cruise vacation.

Vaccines

Regardless of your itinerary, you should be up to date on routine vaccines, such as measles/mumps/rubella, varicella, and seasonal flu. Crew members and fellow travelers often come from countries where these diseases are more common than in the United States and where vaccination is not routine. Consequently, outbreaks of chickenpox and rubella (German measles) have been reported on cruise ships.

Additional vaccines you'll need depend on where you'll be stopping and what you're going to do there. CDC's general vaccination recommendations, by country, can be found on the Travelers'

Health destination pages. However, discuss the cruise itinerary and your specific travel plans with your doctor. If you're stopping in a country only for a short time, or if you don't plan to leave the tourist area around the dock, certain vaccines may not be necessary.

Even if you are not at risk for yellow fever during port calls, some countries in Africa and South America may require proof of yellow fever vaccination if you have previously visited a country with yellow fever. Cruise ship companies sometimes have requirements that differ from those of the countries you will be visiting, so be sure to check with the cruise line about those requirements as well.

Nausea, vomiting, and diarrhea

Cruise ship outbreaks of nausea, vomiting, and diarrhea, primarily caused by norovirus, have been reported. The best way to prevent illness is frequent handwashing with soap and water. Wash your hands before eating and after using the bathroom, changing diapers, or touching things that other people have touched, such as stair railings; it is also a good idea to avoid touching your face.

If soap and water are not available, alcohol-based hand sanitizer (containing at least 60 percent alcohol) is a good second choice. You will see hand sanitizer dispensers throughout your cruise ship—use them.

While on shore excursions, especially in developing countries, follow basic food and water precautions: eat only food that is cooked and served hot, drink only beverages from sealed containers, avoid ice, and eat fresh fruit only if you have washed it with clean water and peeled it yourself.

If you are feeling sick before your voyage, ask your cruise line if alternative cruising options are available. Consult your doctor to find out whether it is safe for you to sail. If you feel sick during your voyage, report your symptoms to the ship's medical facility and follow their recommendations.

Other health concerns

Respiratory diseases are also common on cruise ships. Frequent handwashing can keep you from getting sick, and coughing or sneezing into a tissue (not your hand) can prevent you from spreading germs. Getting a flu shot is the best way to keep from getting the flu.

Seasickness is a common complaint of cruise ship passengers. If you are (or think you might be) prone to seasickness, talk to your doctor about medicine to decrease your symptoms. Note that many common medications (including some antidepressants, painkillers, and birth control pills) can worsen the nausea of seasickness.

Various stressors associated with cruising—changes in diet, variation in climate, changes to sleep and activity patterns—can worsen a chronic illness. If you have been diagnosed with such an illness, you should be prepared to monitor your health while on a cruise (for example, frequently testing your blood sugar if you have diabetes). If you regularly take medicine for a chronic illness, make sure you bring enough for the duration of the cruise, plus extra in case of delays, and take it on the same schedule as you would at home.

For more information on healthy travel, visit www.cdc.gov/travel.

Travel health insurance and evacuation insurance

You should check with your regular health insurance company to see if your policy will cover any medical care you might need in another country or on board the ship. If not, you can purchase travel health insurance to cover you during your trip.

Also, look for gaps in your insurance coverage. For example, your health insurance might not cover medical evacuation if you cannot receive needed treatment where you are. Evacuation by air ambulance can cost $50,000–$100,000 and must be paid in advance by people who do not have insurance. You can buy medical evacuation insurance to be sure you will have access to emergency care.

GETTING SICK AFTER TRAVEL

Feeling ill after your trip? If you went to a country with a Zika outbreak or endemic Zika, you may have the virus. Even if you didn't, you might still have it if you have been sexually exposed to Zika. Although nothing except a positive test can prove you have the illness, looking out for the symptoms of the disease is useful. But remember, around 80 percent of infected people do not have symptoms, so you might feel fine and be carrying the virus. According to the CDC, the symptoms of Zika can include:

Fever
Rash
Joint pain
Conjunctivitis (red eyes)

Other symptoms are:
Muscle pain
Headache

If you get these symptoms, the CDC recommends you "see your doctor or other healthcare provider if you have the symptoms described above and have visited an area with Zika; this is especially important if you are pregnant. Be sure to tell your doctor or other healthcare provider where you traveled."

However, not all fevers are caused by Zika, and sometimes you might suffer from symptoms not on this list. The CDC has identified some of the most common symptoms you may encounter after international travel below. If you're feeling bad, be sure to seek medical attention even if you don't have the symptoms for Zika.

Fever

If you have been in a country with malaria and develop a fever within a month after you leave, see a doctor immediately. Most fevers are caused by less serious illnesses. But because malaria is a medical emergency, your doctor must first rule it out. A fever could still be malaria even if you took antimalarial medicine because the medicine is not 100 percent effective. Most malaria develops within thirty days, but rare cases can lie dormant for a year or longer. So always tell your doctor about any travel you have done, even if it was months ago.

Persistent diarrhea

Most cases of diarrhea go away by themselves in a few days, but see your doctor if you have diarrhea that lasts for two weeks or more. Persistent diarrhea can make you lose nutrients and is often caused by a parasitic infection that will need to be treated with special drugs.

Skin problems

Skin problems (rashes, boils, fungal infections, bug bites) are among the most common illnesses reported by people who have returned from international travel. Most skin problems are not serious, but they may be a sign of a serious illness, especially if you also have a fever.

At the doctor

Whatever the reason, if you go to the doctor after returning from a trip overseas, tell him or her about your recent travel. Make sure to include all relevant details:

- What you did on your trip
- How long you were gone
- Where you stayed (fancy hotel, native dwelling, tent)
- What you ate and drank while you were there
- Whether you were bitten by bugs
- Whether you swam in freshwater
- Any other possible exposures (sex, tattoos, piercings)

ADVENTURE TRAVEL

From the Iguacu National Park to the Amazon River and more, some of the world's greatest adventure tourism sites are located in areas hit by the Zika virus. One of the many reasons tourists are drawn to Zika-prone areas is to engage in adventure tourism. That's why these important CDC guidelines are included to keep you safe on your journey:

Introduction

"Adventure travel" is a type of tourism, often to remote locations, to explore and engage in physical activity. Adventure travel often includes "extreme" activities such as mountain climbing, exploring caves, bungee jumping, mountain biking, rafting, zip-lining, paragliding, and rock climbing.

This fast-growing travel trend is a popular way to see new places and test your physical abilities. However, these activities also present risks to your health and safety. Learning about these risks and preparing for your trip will help make your vacation a fun and safe adventure.

Risks of Adventure Travel

Adventure activities, both at home and abroad, carry some risk of injury. Because this type of international tourism often involves travel to remote locations, additional adventure travel risks include the lack of quick emergency response if injured, poor trauma care, and unexpected weather changes that can make safety challenging and rescue efforts more difficult. Remember that general outdoor risks, such as sunburn and bug bites, apply to adventure travel as well. But most adventure activities can be fun, exciting, *and* safe if you prepare for your trip and follow good safety practices.

Also be aware that if you *are* injured during your trip, your health insurance may not cover health care you receive while abroad. You can buy travel health and evacuation insurance to fill this gap.

What you can do

Adventure travelers, take these steps to prepare for and stay safe during your vacation:

- Make an appointment with a doctor, ideally at least four to six weeks before the trip, to get any recommended vaccinations and medical advice. Be sure to talk to the doctor about your planned adventure activities in case there are special recommendations for you.
- Train properly for your trip. Many adventure tours can be physically demanding, so it is important to be fit before your vacation.

- Check with your regular health insurance company to see if your policy will cover any medical care you might need in another country. If not, consider buying travel health and evacuation insurance.
  - Look for gaps in your insurance coverage. For example, your health insurance might not cover medical evacuation if you cannot receive needed treatment where you are. Evacuation by air ambulance can cost more than $100,000 and must be paid in advance by people who do not have insurance. You can buy medical evacuation insurance to be sure you will have access to emergency care.
  - Evacuation companies often have better resources and experience in some parts of the world than others; travelers may want to ask about a company's resources in a given area before purchase, especially if planning a trip to remote destinations.
- Use a reputable outfitter. Look for a company that has been in business for several years, has a current operating license, and is a member of relevant professional associations such as the local board of tourism. Ask for references and don't be afraid to ask questions!
- Wear protective gear when doing adventure activities and follow safety instructions from your adventure guides.
- Don't drink alcohol before or during outdoor activities.
- Eat and drink regularly to stay hydrated and rest if you feel overheated.
- Avoid too much sun exposure by using sunscreen, wearing protective clothing, and seeking shade.
- Wear bug spray while outdoors to avoid bites from mosquitoes, ticks, and other insects.

- Consider bringing a first aid kit. A number of companies produce advanced medical kits and will customize kits based on specific travel needs.

SEXUAL SAFETY

It is extremely important to protect yourself and your partner from Zika while having sex if you or your partner may have been exposed. With the latest research suggesting that Zika can live in semen for over six months, practicing safe sex and following the appropriate medical advice has never been more crucial. This is particularly important if you are traveling to a Zika-prone location. The CDC has broken down this issue in detail and has the following recommendations:

How Zika is spread through sex

- Zika can be passed through sex from a person with Zika to his or her partners. Sex includes vaginal, anal, and oral sex and the sharing of sex toys.
- Zika can be passed through sex, even if the person does not have symptoms at the time.
  - It can be passed from a person with Zika before their symptoms start, while they have symptoms, and after their symptoms end.
  - Though not well documented, the virus may also be passed by a person who carries the virus but never develops symptoms.

How to protect yourself during sex

- Use condoms and other barriers to protect against infection every time during vaginal, anal, and oral sex.

Barriers that protect against infection include male and female condoms and dental dams. Dental dams are latex or polyurethane sheets used between the mouth and vagina or anus during oral sex.

- Do not share sex toys.
- Not having sex eliminates the risk of getting Zika from sex.

Male Condoms

Condoms are frequently used and well known, but many people don't know the facts about their effectiveness.

In real-life usage, condoms are only 82 percent effective. That number is disturbingly low, given how important condoms are for preventing HIV, syphilis, other STDs, and unplanned pregnancies. But why are they so ineffective?

Because most people use them incorrectly.

In fact, under perfect-use conditions, condoms are 98percent effective. For those engaging in sexual activity with those who have been—or might have been—infected with Zika, condoms are probably your first and perhaps best line of defense. Using condoms without the correct guidelines is like driving a car without a seatbelt—much riskier than it should be. To protect yourself and your partners, these CDC guidelines explain the proper use of condoms:

How to use a condom consistently and correctly

- Use a new condom for every act of vaginal, anal, and oral sex throughout the *entire* sex act (from start to finish). Before any genital contact, put the condom on the tip of the erect penis with the rolled side out.

- If the condom does not have a reservoir tip, pinch the tip enough to leave a half-inch space for semen to collect. Holding the tip, unroll the condom all the way to the base of the erect penis.
- After ejaculation and before the penis gets soft, grip the rim of the condom and carefully withdraw. Then gently pull the condom off the penis, making sure that semen doesn't spill out.
- Wrap the condom in a tissue and throw it in the trash where others won't handle it.
- If you feel the condom break at any point during sexual activity, stop immediately, withdraw, remove the broken condom, and put on a new condom.
- Ensure that adequate lubrication is used during vaginal and anal sex, which might require water-based lubricants. Oil-based lubricants (e.g., petroleum jelly, shortening, mineral oil, massage oils, body lotions, and cooking oil) should not be used because they can weaken latex, causing breakage.

Even if you don't have reason to suspect you or your partner have Zika, there are plenty of good reasons to use condoms. Chlamydia and gonorrhea are common sexually transmitted diseases (STDs) which can result in infertility. Although many people imagine these diseases cause painful sores, often there are no symptoms. These CDC guidelines are helpful reminders of what condoms are protecting you or your partner from:

Chlamydia and gonorrhea are important preventable causes of pelvic inflammatory disease (PID) and infertility. Untreated, about 10–15 percent of women with chlamydia will develop PID. Chlamydia can also cause fallopian tube infection without any symptoms. PID and "silent" infection in the upper genital tract may cause permanent damage to the fallopian tubes, uterus, and surrounding tissues, which can lead to infertility.

- An estimated 2.86 million cases of chlamydia and 820,000 cases of gonorrhea occur annually in the United States.
- Most women infected with chlamydia or gonorrhea have no symptoms.

CDC recommends annual chlamydia and gonorrhea screening of **all sexually active women younger than twenty-five years, as well as older women with risk factors** such as new or multiple sex partners, or a sex partner who has a sexually transmitted infection.

What activities can put me at risk for both STDs and HIV?

- Having anal, vaginal, or oral sex without a condom
- Having multiple sex partners
- Having anonymous sex partners
- Having sex while under the influence of drugs or alcohol can lower inhibitions and result in greater sexual risk-taking.

What can I do to prevent getting STDs and HIV?

The only way to avoid STDs is to not have vaginal, anal, or oral sex. If you are sexually active, you can do the following things to lower your chances of getting STDs and HIV:

- Choose less risky sexual behaviors
- Use condoms consistently and correctly
- Reduce the number of people with whom you have sex

- Limit or eliminate drug and alcohol use before and during sex
- Have an honest and open talk with your healthcare provider and ask whether you should be tested for STDs and HIV
- Talk to your healthcare provider and find out if pre-exposure prophylaxis, or PrEP, is a good option for you to prevent HIV infection

LEGISLATION

Zika funding has been paralyzed by gridlock in Congress. The same political problems and disagreements that led to events like the temporary shutdown of the government have also frozen efforts to pass a $1.1 billion bill to fight Zika.

"So here we are in an utterly absurd position of playing political games as this public health crisis mounts here in our country," said Republican Majority Leader Mitch McConnell on the Senate floor, after the bill was defeated. "Pregnant women all across America are looking at this with dismay, utter dismay, as we sit here in a partisan gridlock manufactured by the other side over issues that it's pretty hard for the general public to understand, refusing to pass the funds needed to address this public health concern."[17]

Senate Minority Leader Harry Reid, had this to say about the bill: "I don't know what universe my friend is living in. What does he think? Does he think we're all stupid? The American people are dumb?"[18] Reid and other Democrats elaborated they were forced to vote against the bill because Republicans packed it with other spending priorities and Republican legislative goals unrelated to the Zika epidemic. Republicans disagreed, leading to continued legislative gridlock and a failure to pass legislation relating to the Zika virus. Many observers believe that the crisis will have to escalate to spur a divided Congress to act. Some believe that no action is likely until after the 2016 presidential elections.

On April 6, 2016, the Obama administration moved $589 million from other sources, including an Ebola fund, towards the Zika epidemic. Shaun Donovan, director of the White House Office of Management and Budget, said, "Nearly two months have passed and the situation continues to grow more critical."[19] In addition to these steps, the Obama administration has also declared Puerto Rico's Zika outbreak a health emergency and allocated extra funds to deal with the situation there. A more lasting and permanent fix has yet to be addressed, and will likely require legislation in Congress.

CDC's Response to **Zika**
ESTIMATED range of *Aedes albopictus* and *Aedes aegypti* in the United States, 2016*

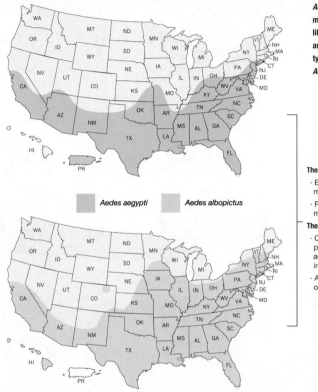

Aedes aegypti mosquitoes are more likely to spread viruses like Zika, dengue, chikungunya and other viruses than other types of mosquitoes such as *Aedes albopictus* mosquitoes.

These maps DO NOT show

· Exact locations or numbers of mosquitoes living in an area

· Risk or likelihood that these mosquitoes will spread viruses

These maps show

· CDC's best estimate of the potential range of *Aedes aegypti* and *Aedes albopictus* in the United States

· Areas where mosquitoes are or have been previously found

Aedes aegypti   *Aedes albopictus*

* Maps have been updated from a variety of sources. These maps represent CDC's best estimate of the potential range of *Aedes aegypti* and *Aedes albopictus* in the United States. Maps are not meant to represent risk for spread of disease.

CS264451-F
April 1, 2016

CDC

U.S. Department of Health and Human Services
Centers for Disease Control and Prevention

Image showing the maximum estimated ranges of *Aedes aegypti* and *Aedes albopictus* mosquitoes.

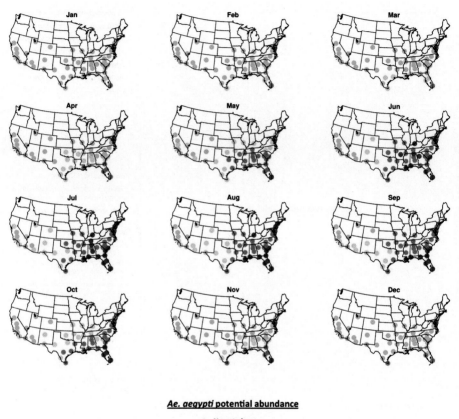

Ae. aegypti potential abundance

- None to low
- Low to moderate
- Moderate to high
- High

The potential prevalence and spread of *Aedes aegypti* mosquitoes by month.

(Monaghan AJ, Morin CW, Steinhoff DF, Wilhelmi O, Hayden M, Quattrochi DA, Reiskind M, Lloyd AL, Smith K, Schmidt CA, Scalf PE, Ernst K. On the Seasonal Occurrence and Abundance of the Zika Virus Vector Mosquito *Aedes Aegypti* in the Contiguous United States. PLOS Currents Outbreaks. 2016 Mar 16. Edition 1. doi: 10.1371/currents. outbreaks.50dfc7f46798675fc63e7d7da563da76.)

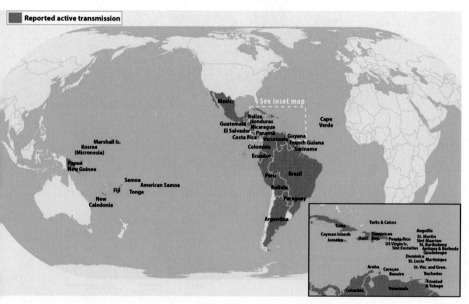

World map including countries with confirmed active transmission of Zika as of early August 2016. Nations shaded in purple have confirmed transmission of the virus.

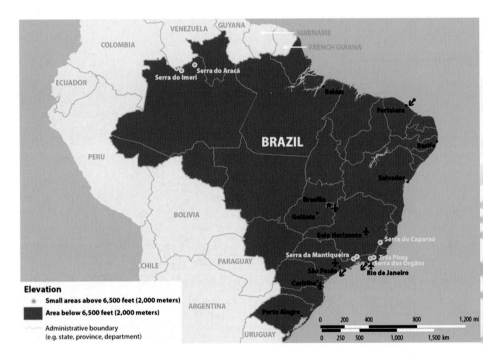

Map of high elevation locations in Brazil. The dark purple locations are low elevation areas, which present the risk of mosquito bites. The light purple areas are high elevation areas, which should have few to no mosquitoes.

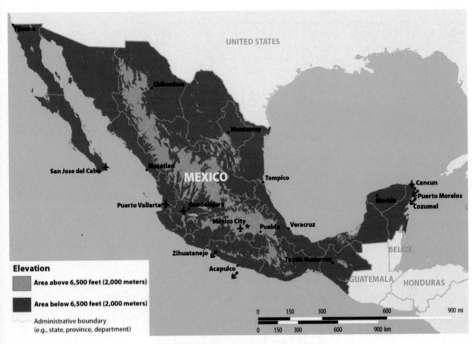

Map of high elevation locations in Mexico. The dark purple locations are low elevation areas, which present the risk of mosquito bites. The light purple areas are high elevation areas, which should have little to no mosquitoes.

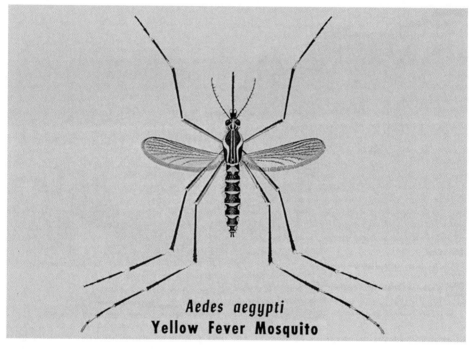

Illustration of the *Aedes aegypti* mosquito.

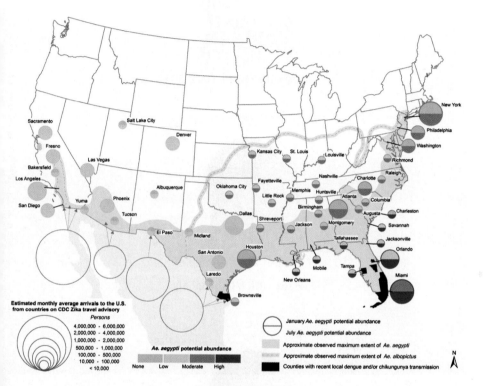

This map looks at travel patterns to the United States from countries with Zika travel advisories to predict where the virus is most likely to spread. The circles show the abundance of *Aeses aegypti* mosquitoes during January (top half of circle) and July (bottom half of circle). The larger the circle, the more arrivals to that location by people from countries on the CDC travel advisory.

(Monaghan AJ, Morin CW, Steinhoff DF, Wilhelmi O, Hayden M, Quattrochi DA, Reiskind M, Lloyd AL, Smith K, Schmidt CA, Scalf PE, Ernst K. On the Seasonal Occurrence and Abundance of the Zika Virus Vector Mosquito *Aedes Aegypti* in the Contiguous United States. PLOS Currents Outbreaks. 2016 Mar 16. Edition 1. doi: 10.1371/currents. outbreaks.50dfc7f46798675fc63e7d7da563da76.)

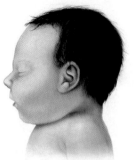

Baby with Typical Head Size

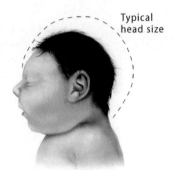

Typical
head size

Baby with Microcephaly

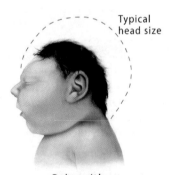

Typical
head size

Baby with
Severe Microcephaly

The effects of microcephaly on the head size of a baby.

5

Getting Zika

SIGNS AND SYMPTOMS

While the initial symptoms of Zika are relatively minor, the long-term effects on yourself or your family are sometimes very serious indeed. What are these symptoms? How long do they last? How can you tell if you have Zika? What tests will doctors use to determine your status? We've answered these and other questions below. First, let's look at the symptoms.

Experiencing the symptoms of Zika is one of the first warnings that you or a loved one may be infected. According to the CDC, the common symptoms of Zika can include:

Fever
Rash
Joint pain
Conjunctivitis (red eyes)

Other symptoms are:
Muscle pain
Headache

These are symptoms common to many illnesses; thus, you should not panic if you experience slight joint pain or a fever, even after visiting a Zika-infected area. However the CDC recommends that you "see your doctor or other healthcare provider if you have the symptoms described above and have visited an area with Zika; this is especially important if you are pregnant. Be sure to tell your doctor or other healthcare provider where you traveled."

Even if you have no symptoms, you can still be infected with Zika. In fact, current estimates suggest around 80 percent of people infected with Zika have no symptoms at all. If you do have symptoms, the CDC has issued information about their severity, and how long the virus usually lasts in the blood.

Zika is usually mild, with symptoms lasting for several days to a week. People usually don't get sick enough to go to the hospital, and they very rarely die of Zika. For this reason, many people might not realize they have been infected. Symptoms of Zika are similar to other viruses spread through mosquito bites, like dengue and chikungunya.

Zika virus usually remains in the blood of an infected person for about a week. See your doctor or other healthcare provider if you develop symptoms and you live in or have recently traveled to an area with Zika. Your doctor or other healthcare provider may order blood tests to look for Zika or other similar viruses like dengue or chikungunya. Once a person has been infected, he or she is likely to be protected from future infections.

TREATING THE INITIAL SYMPTOMS OF ZIKA

If you experience the symptoms above and have been to a Zika-infected area, talking to your doctor is the best first step. To treat your symptoms, taking drugs that contain acetaminophen—such as Tylenol—may help lessen the pain or discomfort you are feeling. Tylenol is perhaps the most well-known drug with acetaminophen sold in the United States; however, a generic drug with acetaminophen will work just as well. Tylenol and generic alternatives can be found at nearly any drugstore in the United

States, and at many gas stations, grocery stores, and other shops. However, if you are traveling abroad, you may get a confused look if you ask a local shopkeeper for Tylenol. That's because outside of the United States, the naming conventions for the drug are somewhat different.

In some foreign countries, acetaminophen is instead known as paracetamol. Despite the naming difference, the drug is the same. Moreover, while Tylenol is the most well-known brand name for acetaminophen in the United States, in many foreign countries the brand name Panadol is more popular. As with any medicine, there are risks and side effects of acetaminophen. In particular, the use of alcohol and acetaminophen should be avoided. Special care should be taken when administering the drug to children. Be sure to carefully read the instructions and consult your doctor if you have any questions.

What about other painkillers?

Although acetaminophen may help take the edge off, you will want to avoid painkillers like Motrin, Advil, and aspirin, or any drug that contains aspirin, ibuprofen, or naproxen, because they are blood thinners. These drugs are also known collectively as NSAIDs (nonsteroidal anti-inflammatory drugs). Taking these drugs could potentially be dangerous if you are actually infected with dengue instead of Zika.

IS IT DENGUE?

If you've been in a Zika-infected area, you may have been bitten by the *Aedes aegypti* mosquito. This mosquito not only spreads Zika, but also dengue fever, a different disease. According to the CDC, "Zika and dengue virus share similar symptoms of infection, transmission cycles, and geographic distribution."

If you actually have dengue instead of Zika, taking NSAIDs could be deadly. Dengue affects blood platelets, making it harder for blood to form clots and stop bleeding. NSAIDs also retard blood clotting, making those who are actually infected with dengue who also take NSAIDs susceptible to dangerous levels of bleeding.

However, the symptoms of dengue are usually more severe than Zika. The CDC has identified these symptoms of dengue, and issued advice for those who may be suffering from it:

High fever *and* at least two of the following:

- Severe headache
- Severe eye pain (behind eyes)
- Joint pain
- Muscle and/or bone pain
- Rash
- Mild bleeding manifestation (e.g., nose or gum bleed, petechiae, or easy bruising)
- Low white cell count

Generally, younger children and those with their first dengue infection have a milder illness than older children and adults.

Watch for warning signs as temperature declines three to seven days after symptoms began.

Go **IMMEDIATELY** to an emergency room or the closest health care provider if any of the following *warning signs* appear:

- Severe abdominal pain or persistent vomiting
- Red spots or patches on the skin
- Bleeding from nose or gums

- Vomiting blood
- Black, tarry stools
- Drowsiness or irritability
- Pale, cold, or clammy skin
- Difficulty breathing

If you are experiencing these symptoms, or have other reasons to believe you may have dengue, be sure to follow the CDC's advice and see a doctor or go to the emergency room immediately. Dengue is a serious disease that requires professional medical attention.

TESTING

Doctors and medical professionals currently have several testing options to determine whether a patient has Zika. Some of the most popular tests include the rRT-PCR test, the Zika MAC-ELISA test, and the PRNT test. Others are constantly being developed and refined, and may be available from a healthcare professional.

Who should get tested?

Consult a medical professional who will be able to help you decide whether a Zika test is right for you. Remember, although stories about Zika in the news may be frightening, the impact for most Americans is likely to be limited. If you live in a cold-weather state or it is winter, you are unlikely to be at risk of mosquito bites. If you are not engaged in a sexual relationship with someone who is at risk of Zika transmission, or you are practicing safe sex with condoms or other blocking contraceptives, your risk is also likely to be low.

Those who have visited or live in a location with epidemic or endemic Zika, or are engaged in a sexual relationship with someone who has, or have other reasons to believe they may have Zika should contact a healthcare professional to determine whether a Zika test is a smart choice. There are currently no widely available home-based testing options, although these are currently in development.

TYPES OF TESTS

The shocking spread of the Zika virus has meant that the medical community has rushed to make Zika tests available. New tests and ways of detecting the virus are constantly being developed. For now, these are the three most common ways that medical professionals determine whether you have Zika:

rRT-PCR Test

How it works: The rRT-PCR test looks for Zika RNA—a type of genetic material—in blood serum or urine samples.

Time frame: The rRT-PCR blood test may be able to detect Zika RNA within around one week of infection.

The rRT-PCR urine test can also identify Zika within around two weeks of infection.

Samples required: Blood, urine.

One popular method is the rRT-PCR test. An acronym for real-time reverse transcription-polymerase chain reaction, this test can identify Zika virus's genetic material in blood serum or urine.

While it is a good test, there are several caveats to be aware of. First, it is only effective at finding Zika in blood serum samples during approximately the first five to seven days after an infection. That means patients—and doctors—need to act quickly if this test is to be effective. Luckily, the telltale signs of Zika survive longer in urine, up to around two weeks, giving professionals a longer window to diagnose the disease.

According to the CDC, "a positive rRT-PCR result on any sample confirms Zika virus infection and no additional testing is indicated." However, "A negative rRT-PCR result does not exclude Zika virus infection" and further testing will be necessary to determine whether you are infected with Zika. If you tested negative for Zika using the rRT-PCR test, or simply waited too long, you may be referred to another popular test, known as the Zika MAC-ELISA.

Zika MAC-ELISA

How it works: The Zika Mac-ELISA test looks for antibodies produced in response to a Zika infection.

Time frame: This test can detect Zika up to twelve weeks after infection, and perhaps longer.

Samples required: Blood or cerebrospinal fluid (CSF)

Described by NPR as the "the best test available right now,"[20] the CDC has laid out important information about the use of the MAC-ELISA test, some of which is excerpted here.

The Zika MAC-ELISA is a laboratory test to detect proteins the human body makes to fight a Zika virus infection. These proteins, called antibodies, appear in the blood starting four to five days after the start of illness and last for up to twelve weeks. In some people, they are present for longer than twelve weeks.

If you have a positive result with the Zika MAC-ELISA, it is likely that you recently were infected with the Zika virus. There is a chance that this test can give a positive result that is wrong; this is called a false positive result. There are some other very closely related viruses (such as dengue virus) that can cause the human body to produce antibodies that may cause the test to be positive. If your result from this test is positive or equivocal (unclear), you should ask your healthcare provider or health department if additional testing has or will be carried out to rule out a false positive result. It is important that you work with your healthcare provider or health department to help you understand the next steps you should take.

If you have a negative test, it does not necessarily mean that you have not been infected with Zika virus. If your sample was collected just after you became ill, it is possible that your body had not yet had enough time to make antibodies for the test to measure. If the sample was collected more than twelve weeks after your illness, it is possible that your body has already fought off the virus and the amount of antibodies is so low that they cannot be measured. Your healthcare provider will help you to interpret your test results and work with you to continue to monitor your health.

At the time of this writing, the CDC has noted, "The Zika MAC-ELISA has not been cleared or approved by the US Food and Drug Administration (FDA). However, FDA has authorized the emergency use of this test under an Emergency Use Authorization (EUA)." This is because "there are no FDA approved/cleared alternative tests available that detect Zika virus infection. FDA has authorized the emergency use of the Zika MAC-ELISA to test for antibodies to Zika virus in blood and CSF. Use of this test is authorized only for the duration of the potential emergency, unless it is terminated or revoked by FDA sooner." Check with your healthcare provider or the CDC website (cdc.gov/zika) for the latest information on the status of the Zika MAC-ELISA test.

PRNT

How it works: The PRNT (plaque-reduction neutralization test)
Time frame: This test can detect Zika up to twelve weeks after infection, and perhaps longer.
Samples required: Blood or cerebrospinal fluid (CSF)

The PRNT test is another important test doctors use to determine whether you are infected with Zika. While it is quite accurate, it takes several days longer than other tests. To do this test, the Zika virus is grown in human cells in a laboratory, and then exposed to the patient's blood sample. If the patient has been exposed to Zika before, they should have antibodies in their blood, which will inhibit the growth of the Zika virus.

To test this, the blood and Zika virus mixture is placed on a fresh set of cells, and scientists track the growth. If the patient has been exposed to Zika before, the virus should be at least somewhat inhibited after exposure to the antibodies. If they have not been exposed, there should be no inhibition and the virus will grow freely. Depending on the amount of growth inhibited, the time frame in which the patient contracted Zika can be estimated.

If you have received a positive result in another Zika test, this one may not be necessary. Furthermore, the testing guidelines may quickly change as new tests and methods are brought to market. Check the CDC's website at cdc.gov/zika, or consult your healthcare provider for the latest information.

DIAGNOSIS

Multiple tests may be required to determine whether you have Zika. Some tests may not be able to easily distinguish between Zika and other similar viruses like dengue. Regardless of whether your test results were positive, negative, or inconclusive, be sure to stay calm and focus on putting your health first. Learning that you or a loved one may be infected by Zika is not a pleasant experience, but by focusing on treatment and asking medical professionals for the best, most up-to-date advice, you can focus on the important part: getting better.

Positive test results and pregnancy

If you are pregnant and have received a positive test result, don't panic. Not all pregnant women who test positive for Zika will have babies that develop birth defects or other problems. The CDC notes:

Studies have reported that some, but not all, babies born to women with positive Zika test results during pregnancy were born with microcephaly and other problems. At this time, we do not know how often a baby will have microcephaly or other problems if a woman is infected with Zika while she is pregnant. Your doctor or other healthcare provider will watch your pregnancy more closely if you have a positive Zika virus test. This test can also give positive results when the patient has had an infection with a virus other than Zika virus. The results of this test are not conclusive—a positive test result for Zika virus infection during pregnancy signals to your doctor or other healthcare provider to watch your pregnancy more closely, meaning he or she might do more ultrasounds or other tests to check the growth and development of your fetus and check for any signs of Zika virus infection.

This topic is also covered in the following chapter.

What to do if you are infected

If you learn you have been infected with Zika, don't panic. Your doctor and other healthcare professionals will work with you to develop a treatment plan to deal with the virus. Prevention, covered in the previous chapter, will be key to protecting your family, loved ones, and your community from a further spread of the virus.

Perhaps the only bright side of contracting Zika is that, once you have it, you are unlikely to ever catch it again. After you have recovered from your initial infection, antibodies will likely protect you from further infections. If you are not a pregnant woman or a woman likely to soon become pregnant, the threat Zika poses is relatively low. Most symptoms will fade within a week. If you have contracted the virus, remember that while your symptoms may have faded, the virus can still be present in your blood or other bodily fluids. Taking care not to infect your loved ones or sexual partners is key.

TREATMENT

There is no cure for Zika, but the symptoms can be mitigated. As mentioned earlier, taking acetaminophen should help alleviate any pain or discomfort you may feel. Focusing on rest and staying hydrated is important, as it will give your body time to heal. Be sure you have ruled out dengue before taking NSAIDs like Motrin or aspirin, which could result in excessive bleeding.

The most important treatment for anyone suffering from Zika is rest, water, and a strict focus on prevention to make sure that others around you do not get the virus. While there may not yet be a cure for Zika, you should do all you can to make sure that your loved ones, your community, and those around you do not contract the virus.

6

Pregnancy and Birth Control

RISK OF EXPOSURE

Anyone who travels to a Zika-prone area or has sexual contact with someone infected with the virus is at risk for Zika. Although local transmission of the virus in the continental United States is currently restricted to southern Florida, this is likely to change. In fact, as the virus continues to spread, it is likely that larger swaths of the United States will be home to Zika-carrying mosquitoes. Millions of people across the world are already at risk of the virus, and one estimate suggests a total of 2.2 billion people could be at risk. The WHO has estimated that around three to four million people are likely to be infected by the end of 2016.

While being exposed to Zika is troubling for any person, current evidence suggests that symptoms and side effects are generally minor, although a small percentage of adults will suffer from GBS after contracting Zika. However, pregnant women and those likely to become pregnant suffer greater risk given the correlation between Zika and microcephaly. Because microcephaly is a serious condition that can result in permanent disabilities for the afflicted children, pregnant women must take extra precautions.

Although pregnant women face extra risks, they are not any more susceptible to catching the virus. If you are pregnant or planning to become pregnant, you should avoid travel to Zika-prone locations unless absolutely necessary. If you live in an area with Zika or have an infected partner, you should follow these CDC guidelines to minimize your risk of infection.

PRECAUTIONARY MEASURES

The precautionary measures for pregnant women are the same as for all other people, although given the potential consequences of microcephaly, pregnant women should exercise extreme care to prevent infection by Zika. The CDC has specific advice for avoiding Zika infection, which is included below. Women traveling to foreign countries that are experiencing Zika outbreaks should consult this book's section on foreign travel for even more information.

Everyone living in or traveling to areas with Zika should take steps to prevent mosquito bites:

- Cover exposed skin by wearing long-sleeved shirts and long pants.
- Use EPA-registered insect repellents that contain one of the following active ingredients: DEET, picaridin, IR3535, or oil of lemon eucalyptus or para-menthane-diol. Always use as directed.
  - Pregnant and breastfeeding women can use all EPA-registered insect repellents according to the product label.
  - Most repellents can be used on children older than two months old. To apply, adults should spray insect repellent onto hands and then apply to a child's face.
    - Do not use products containing oil of lemon eucalyptus (OLE) or para-menthane-diol (PMD) on children under three years old.

- Use permethrin-treated clothing and gear (boots, pants, socks, tents). You can buy pre-treated items or treat them yourself.
- Stay and sleep in screened-in or air-conditioned rooms.
- Sleep under a mosquito bed net if air-conditioned or screened rooms are not available or if sleeping outdoors.
- Mosquito netting can be used to cover babies younger than two months old in carriers, strollers, or cribs to protect them from mosquito bites.
- Take steps to control mosquitoes in and around your home.

PREVENTING THE SEXUAL TRANSMISSION OF ZIKA

Even if you are not visiting or living in an area with active Zika transmission, you might still be vulnerable to the sexual spread of the virus. That's why understanding your birth control options is so important.

All types of birth control are designed to prevent pregnancy, but not all types of birth control can prevent the sexual spread of Zika.

If you believe your partner may have Zika, it is best to choose a birth control option like the male condom that can both prevent pregnancy and also prevent the sexual spread of Zika. Theoretically, a birth control method that merely prevents pregnancy but does not prevent the spread of Zika—like the pill—will also protect against microcephaly, given that there will be no baby to contract the condition. However, this is not the safest and most responsible course of action. Birth control sometimes fails, and if you have recently contracted Zika and become pregnant, your baby will be at risk.

We still do not know the long-term effects of the virus, although it is believed that women who have contracted Zika and recovered will, in the vast majority of cases, give birth to babies without microcephaly. Since Zika can result in Guillain-Barré syndrome, avoiding infection is your best bet regardless of whether you are taking other birth control that will prevent pregnancy. The CDC has noted:

Condoms (and other barriers to protect against infection) can reduce the chance of getting Zika from sex. To be effective, condoms should be used from start to finish every time during vaginal, anal, and oral sex. It can be passed from a person with Zika before their symptoms start, while they have symptoms, and after their symptoms end.

- All pregnant women with sex partners who live in or have traveled to an area with Zika should use condoms or not have sex during their pregnancy, even if their partners do not have Zika symptoms, or if their symptoms have gone away.
- Couples who traveled to the area can consider using condoms or not having sex for at least eight weeks after travel.
- Anyone concerned about sexual transmission of Zika can consider using condoms or not having sex while there is Zika in the area.

BIRTH CONTROL: OVERVIEW

As the most serious risks of Zika affect pregnant women and their unborn children, many women worried about Zika are considering delaying pregnancies to be safe. After all, your child can't suffer from microcephaly if he or she hasn't been conceived yet. While abstaining from sexual activity is one option, many people opt to use birth control instead. This section looks at all major types of birth control, explaining how they work, what the benefits are, and the various pros and cons of each way of preventing an unplanned pregnancy.

Reversible birth control methods: An overview

If you're thinking about birth control, it pays to understand your options. The following CDC list includes all commonly used reversible methods of birth control. Nonreversible methods are covered next.

Intrauterine contraception

- **Copper T intrauterine device (IUD)**: This IUD is a small device that is shaped in the form of a "T." Your doctor places it inside the uterus to prevent pregnancy. It can stay in your uterus for up to ten years. Typical use failure rate: 0.8 percent. Women can have the Copper T IUD inserted within five days of unprotected sex.
- **Levonorgestrel intrauterine system (LNG IUD)**: The LNG IUD is a small T-shaped device like the Copper T IUD. It is placed inside the uterus by a doctor. It releases a small amount of progestin each day to keep you from getting pregnant. The LNG IUD stays in your uterus for up to five years. Typical use failure rate: 0.2 percent.

Hormonal Methods

- **Implant**: The implant is a single thin rod that is inserted under the skin of a women's upper arm. The rod contains a progestin that is released into the body over three years. Typical use failure rate: 0.05 percent.

- **Injection or "shot"**: Women get shots of the hormone progestin in the buttocks or arm every three months from their doctor. Typical use failure rate: 6 percent.
- **Combined oral contraceptives**: Also called "the pill," combined oral contraceptives contain the hormones estrogen and progestin. It is prescribed by a doctor. A pill is taken at the same time each day. If you are thirty-five or older and smoke, have a history of blood clots or breast cancer, your doctor may advise you not to take the pill. Typical use failure rate: 9 percent.
- **Progestin-only pill**: Unlike the combined pill, the progestin-only pill (sometimes called the mini-pill) only has one hormone, progestin, instead of both estrogen and progestin. It is prescribed by a doctor. It is taken at the same time each day. It may be a good option for women who can't take estrogen. Typical use failure rate: 9 percent.
- **Patch**: This skin patch is worn on the lower abdomen, buttocks, or upper body (but not on the breasts). This method is prescribed by a doctor. It releases hormones progestin and estrogen into the bloodstream. You put on a new patch once a week for three weeks. During the fourth week, you do not wear a patch, so you can have a menstrual period. Typical use failure rate: 9 percent, but may be higher in women who weigh more than 198 pounds.
- **Hormonal vaginal contraceptive ring**: The ring releases the hormones progestin and estrogen. You place the ring inside your vagina. You wear the ring for three weeks, take it out for the week you have your period, and then put in a new ring. Typical use failure rate: 9 percent.

- **Emergency contraception**: Emergency contraception is *not* a regular method of birth control. Emergency contraception can be used after no birth control was used during sex, or if the birth control method failed, such as if a condom broke. Women can take emergency contraceptive pills up to five days after unprotected sex, but the sooner the pills are taken, the better they will work. There are three different types of emergency contraceptive pills available in the United States. Some emergency contraceptive pills are available over the counter.

Barrier Methods

- **Diaphragm or cervical cap**: Each of these barrier methods are placed inside the vagina to cover the cervix to block sperm. The diaphragm is shaped like a shallow cup. The cervical cap is a thimble-shaped cup. Before sexual intercourse, you insert them with spermicide to block or kill sperm. Visit your doctor for a proper fitting because diaphragms and cervical caps come in different sizes. Typical use failure rate: 12 percent.
- **Male condom**: Worn by the man, a condom keeps sperm from getting into a woman's body. Latex condoms, the most common type, help prevent pregnancy and HIV and other STDs, as do the newer synthetic condoms. "Natural" or "lambskin" condoms also help prevent pregnancy, but may not provide protection against STDs, including HIV. Typical use failure rate: 18 percent. Condoms can only be used once. You can buy condoms, KY jelly, or water-based lubricants at a drugstore. Do not use oil-based lubricants such as massage oils, baby oil,

lotions, or petroleum jelly with latex condoms. They will weaken the condom, causing it to tear or break.

- **Female condom**: Worn by the woman, the female condom helps keeps sperm from getting into her body. It is packaged with a lubricant and is available at drugstores. It can be inserted up to eight hours before sexual intercourse. Typical use failure rate: 21 percent, and also may help prevent STDs.
- **Spermicides**: These products work by killing sperm and come in several forms—foam, gel, cream, film, suppository, or tablet. They are placed in the vagina no more than one hour before intercourse. You leave them in place at least six to eight hours after intercourse. You can use a spermicide in addition to a male condom, diaphragm, or cervical cap. They can be purchased at drugstores. Typical use failure rate: 28 percent.

Fertility Awareness-Based Methods

- **Natural family planning or fertility awareness**: Understanding your monthly fertility pattern can help you plan to get pregnant or avoid getting pregnant. Your fertility pattern is the number of days in the month when you are fertile (able to get pregnant), days when you are infertile, and days when fertility is unlikely, but possible. If you have a regular menstrual cycle, you have about nine or more fertile days each month. If you do not want to get pregnant, you do not have sex on the days you are fertile, or you use a barrier method of birth control on those days. Failure rates vary across these methods. Overall, typical use failure rate: 24 percent.

Permanent Birth Control Methods: An Overview

Although most people using birth control opt for reversible methods, if you are certain that you do not want to conceive a child in the future, these methods, covered by the CDC below, are a potential option. Remember, even if you are unable to become pregnant, in the absence of blocking birth control like condoms, or abstaining from sex entirely, you may still contract the Zika virus from sex. However, microcephaly will not be a problem, as it only strikes developing fetuses.

Contraceptive sterilization is a permanent, safe, and highly effective approach for birth control. These methods are meant for people who are sure that they do not desire a pregnancy in the future.

The following methods have a typical use failure rate of less than 1 percent.

- **Female Sterilization, Tubal Ligation or "tying tubes"**: A woman can have her fallopian tubes tied (or closed) so that sperm and eggs cannot meet for fertilization. The procedure can be done in a hospital or in an outpatient surgical center. You can go home the same day of the surgery and resume your normal activities within a few days. This method is effective immediately.
- **Transcervical Sterilization**: A thin tube is used to thread a tiny device into each fallopian tube. It irritates the fallopian tubes and causes scar tissue to grow and permanently plug the tubes. It can take about three months for the scar tissue to grow, so use another form of birth control during this time. Return to your doctor for a test to see if scar tissue has fully blocked your fallopian tubes.

- **Male Sterilization, Vasectomy**: This operation is done to keep a man's sperm from going to his penis, so his ejaculate never has any sperm in it that can fertilize an egg. The procedure is done at an outpatient surgical center. The man can go home the same day. Recovery time is less than one week. After the operation, a man visits his doctor for tests to count his sperm and to make sure the sperm count has dropped to zero; this takes about twelve weeks. Another form of birth control should be used until the man's sperm count has dropped to zero.

Although most women and men who undergo contraceptive sterilization do not regret having had the procedure, the permanence of the method is an important consideration, as regret has been documented in studies. For example, the US Collaborative Review of Sterilization (CREST) study found that women who were younger at the time of the procedure were more likely to experience regret.

An additional issue addressed by the CREST study was the question of whether women who underwent contraceptive sterilization developed a "post-tubal ligation syndrome" of menstrual abnormalities, something that had been debated for years. Results indicated that menstrual abnormalities were no more common among women who had undergone tubal sterilization than among women who had not.

When considering a vasectomy, it's important to understand that failures can occur. CDC research has estimated there is a probability of eleven failures per 1,000 procedures over two years; half of the failures occurred in the first three months after the vasectomy, and no failures occurred after seventy-two weeks. CDC research also examined regret among women whose partner underwent a vasectomy. In interviews with female partners of men who received vasectomies, CDC found that while most women did not regret their husband's vasectomies, the probability of regret over five years was about 6 percent. This is why it is important to know facts about this and other permanent forms of birth control before making a decision.

BIRTH CONTROL IN DEPTH: THE PILL

Will prevent pregnancy, but will not protect against Zika virus transmission.

Oral contraceptives, commonly known as "the pill," are a popular way for women to prevent or delay pregnancy. While the pill is effective at preventing pregnancy, it will not protect against the spread of sexually transmitted diseases, HIV, or Zika. However, if you are not pregnant, you won't be able to give birth to a baby with microcephaly. Thus, if you expect you may be at risk for any of these risk factors, or are engaged in sexual activity with a new partner, you may want to combine use of the pill with condoms, or abstain from sexual activity altogether. The CDC has multiple guidelines and information related to the pill, which is excerpted in part here:

What is the birth control pill?

The birth control pill, also known as oral contraceptives or just "the pill," is a medication taken daily to prevent pregnancy. Some women take the pill for reasons other than preventing pregnancy.

Combined pills contain two hormones, estrogen and progestin. Hormones are chemicals that control how different parts of your body work. These pills are taken every day and prevent pregnancy by keeping the ovaries from releasing eggs. The pills also cause cervical mucus to thicken and the lining of the uterus to thin. This keeps sperm from meeting with and fertilizing an egg.

Progestin-only pills (or "mini-pills") contain only one hormone, progestin, which causes cervical mucus to thicken and the lining of the uterus to thin. This keeps sperm from reaching the egg. Less often, mini-pills prevent pregnancy by keeping the ovaries from releasing eggs.

How do I use it?

Combined pills are typically packaged as twenty-one "active" pills that contain hormones. One pill is taken daily for three weeks, followed by one week off. Others are packaged as twenty-eight pills that include twenty-one "active" pills taken daily, followed by one week of "inactive" reminder pills that don't contain hormones.

Some newer formulations have increased the number of active pills to twenty-four and reduced the inactive pills to four. With all combined pill formulations, protection against pregnancy continues during the week where no active pills are taken.

Some women use combined pills to limit the number of periods they have, or even to prevent them altogether:

- *Extended Cycle* use involves taking twelve weeks of active pills followed by one week of inactive pills. Women on an extended cycle have three or four periods a year.
- *Continuous Use* of pills is where a woman takes an active pill every day so she won't have any periods at all.

Mini-pills come only in packages of twenty-eight–day "active" pills. It is important to take mini-pills every day, and to take them at the **same time** each day. If you're late taking a mini-pill by more than three hours, you'll need to use another type of birth control (such as a condom or sponge) to prevent pregnancy, but continue also to take the mini-pill.

All types of birth control pills should be taken **exactly** as directed by your health care provider, even on days when you don't have sex.

Effectiveness in preventing pregnancy

- Of 100 women who use this method each year, about nine may get pregnant.
- The risk is lower in women who take birth control pills correctly—every day at about the same time.

Advantages of the pill

- The pill is easy to use.
- Birth control pills are safe and work well in preventing pregnancy. Using the pill means you don't have to think about birth control when you want to have sex.
- Combination pills may offer other benefits such as fewer menstrual cramps, decreased menstrual blood loss, less acne, and stronger bones. They also reduce the risk of some cancers that affect reproductive organs.
- Fertility returns to normal when women discontinue use.

Drawbacks of the pill

- The pill does not protect against sexually transmitted infections (STIs), including HIV.

- You need to visit a healthcare provider to get a prescription.
- You must take your pills every day.
- Certain medications such as Rifampin (taken to treat tuberculosis) and supplements (such as St. John's Wort) may make the pill less effective.
- Combined pills may cause nausea, changes in your menstrual cycle, breast tenderness, or headaches. Discuss your medical history with your healthcare provider before using any birth control pill, and let them know if you develop any side effects.
- It is uncommon, but some women develop high blood pressure.
- Rarely, use of the combined pill increases the risk of blood clots, heart attack, and stroke. The risk of blood clots increases for very overweight women who use the combined pill.

How do I get it?

You need a prescription from your healthcare provider. Birth control pills can be purchased at pharmacies or obtained from a health center, including a family planning center. To find a family planning center near you visit www.hhs.gov/opa.

Be sure to consult your medical professional when deciding what type of birth control may be right for you and your partner.

BIRTH CONTROL IN DEPTH: MALE CONDOMS

Prevents pregnancy and transmission of the Zika virus when used effectively.

Male condoms are a popular and commonly used way to prevent pregnancy and the spread of STDs. The CDC has issued a wealth of information on their benefits, drawbacks, and tips for proper use, some of which is excerpted below:

What is the male condom?

A male condom is a thin film sheath that's placed over the penis. Condoms prevent pregnancy by keeping sperm from entering a woman's body.

Condoms—sometimes called "rubbers"—made from latex rubber are the most common type. For people who get skin irritation from latex, polyurethane condoms are a good choice.

Condoms come either lubricated or non-lubricated. You can also add water-based lubricant, such as KY jelly, to a condom to make sex more comfortable. Avoid oil-based lubricants (e.g., petroleum jelly, massage oil, body lotion) as these weaken condoms and may cause them to break.

Used correctly each time you have sex, latex and polyurethane condoms do a good job of preventing pregnancy and many sexually transmitted infections (STIs). Condoms made from natural or lambskin materials also protect against pregnancy, but they won't protect against some STIs.

How do I use it?

- Put a condom on the erect penis before sex.
- To keep semen from spilling, pull the penis out before it gets soft.
- Hold the condom against the base of the penis when pulling out.
- Use the condom once and then throw it away.

Condoms can be damaged by heat, so store them somewhere cool and dry. Don't store them in a wallet or in a car.

Advantages of the male condom

- You don't need a prescription.
- Anyone can buy them.
- Male condoms are safe and easy to use.
- They can be used for vaginal, anal, and oral sex. Ask for flavored condoms to improve the experience when using them for protection against STIs with oral sex.
- Latex and polyurethane condoms offer protection against STIs, including HIV, as well as pregnancy.

Drawbacks of the male condom

- You must use a new condom each time you have sex.
- Condoms made from latex can cause irritation or allergic reactions in some people.
- A male partner has to agree to use male condoms.

How effective are male condoms?

Of 100 couples each year whose partners use male condoms, about eighteen women may get pregnant. Condoms are more effective at preventing pregnancy when they are used correctly and when you use them every time you have sex.

How do I get male condoms?

You can buy condoms at many stores, including pharmacies and grocery and discount stores. Health departments, clinics, and student health centers may offer free or low-cost condoms. You do not need a prescription or an ID to buy them.

To search for a family planning center near you, go to www. hhs.gov/opa.

BIRTH CONTROL IN DEPTH: THE PATCH

Prevents pregnancy, but will not protect against Zika virus transmission.

The patch is another commonly used form of birth control, popular because it allows a woman to simply place a patch on her skin, instead of having to take pills or get shots. Although it is effective at preventing pregnancy, it will not prevent against the sexual spread of Zika. The CDC has offered information on the patch, how it should be used, and what the benefits and drawbacks of this birth control method are. Some of this information is excerpted below:

What is the birth control patch?

The birth control patch is a thin, beige plastic square about two inches across that looks like a Band-Aid. It contains progestin and estrogen—hormones found in most birth control pills. Hormones are chemicals that control how different parts of your body work. The patch has a sticky side that can be attached to the skin of the stomach, buttocks, back or upper outer arm.

The hormones in the patch are absorbed into the bloodstream through the skin and prevent pregnancy by keeping the ovaries from releasing eggs. The patch also causes cervical mucus to thicken and the lining of the uterus to thin. This keeps sperm from meeting and fertilizing the egg.

The patch is sold under the brand name Ortho Evra.

How do I use it?

You put a new patch on each week for three weeks (take off the old patch and throw it away). During the fourth week, you do not wear a patch and your period will probably start. After the fourth week, start over again and put on a new patch (even if there is still some bleeding from your period).

- To help you remember, try to put a new patch on the same day each week.
- Put the patch on clean, dry skin and press to make sure it will stay on. Be careful not to touch the sticky side while putting it on your skin.
- Look each day to make sure the patch is still in place.
- It is okay to bathe and swim while wearing a patch.
- It is better not to place the patch on a breast.
- If the patch comes loose or falls off, you may need to use another method of birth control, like a condom.

Discuss your medical history with your health care provider before using the patch and let him/her know if you develop any side effects.

Advantages of the patch

- Easy to use and does not require the consent of a partner.
- Safe and works well to prevent pregnancy. Using the patch means you do not have to think about birth control when you want to have sex.
- You can see the patch and be reassured it's still there.
- May make your periods lighter and more regular.
- May reduce menstrual cramps and acne, and strengthen bones.
- Reduces the risk of developing non-cancerous breast tumors and some cancers that affect reproductive organs.

Drawbacks of the patch

- Does not protect against sexually transmitted infections (STIs), including HIV.

- Requires a visit to a healthcare provider and a prescription.
- Certain medications such as Rifampin (taken to treat tuberculosis) and supplements (such as St. John's Wort) may make the patch less effective.
- It may take a month or two after stopping the patch before normal periods return.
- Some women experience skin irritation where the patch is worn. Others may have breast tenderness.
- It exposes users to higher levels of estrogen compared to most combined oral contraceptives (birth control pills).
- It is not known if serious risks, such as blood clots and strokes, are greater with the patch than with birth control pills and the vaginal ring due to the greater exposure to estrogen.

How effective is it?

- Of 100 women who use this method each year, about nine may get pregnant.

The risk of pregnancy is much less for women who use the patch correctly (putting it on the skin the same time each week). The patch may be less effective in women who weigh more than one hundred ninety-eight pounds. Certain medications such as Rifampin (taken to treat tuberculosis) and supplements (such as St. John's Wort) may make the patch less effective.

Talk with your healthcare provider if you have any questions about using the patch.

How do I get it?

You need a prescription. The patch can be purchased at pharmacies and is also available at some health centers. To search for a family planning center near you, go to www.hhs.gov/opa.

BIRTH CONTROL IN DEPTH:
EMERGENCY CONTRACEPTION

Prevents pregnancy after sex, but will not protect against Zika transmission.

Emergency contraception is a type of birth control that can be used after sexual intercourse. While it can prevent pregnancy if used quickly enough, it cannot prevent the sexual spread of the Zika virus. If you believe you may have Zika and recently engaged in unprotected sex, emergency contraception may be a good choice for you. After all, if you're not pregnant, you can't deliver birth to a baby with microcephaly. The CDC has issued a wealth of information on this important form of birth control, much of which is included below.

What is emergency contraception?

Emergency contraception is birth control that you use *after* you have had unprotected sex—if you didn't use birth control or your regular birth control failed. Depending on the type of emergency contraception, you can use emergency contraception within three days or within five days after unprotected sex to prevent pregnancy.

There are two types of emergency contraception (EC):

1. Emergency contraceptive pills (ECPs)
a. *Plan B One-Step, Next Choice One Dose,* and *My Way* consist of one pill that the instructions state must be taken with three days (seventy-two hours).
b. *Levonorgestrel Tablets* consist of two pills. Although the instructions state that the first one must be taken within three days (seventy-two hours) and another must be taken twelve hours later, both pills can be

taken at the same time within four days (ninety-six hours) after unprotected sex.

c. *ella* consists of one pill that must be taken within five days (120 hours).

Research has shown that the pills in a and b above are equally effective when taken on the first-fourth days after unprotected sex and are ineffective thereafter. ella is equally effective when taken on the first-fifth days.

2. Emergency insertion of a copper T intrauterine device (IUD) within five days (120 hours)

How do I use it?

Emergency contraception is birth control that you use after you have had unprotected sex—if you did not use birth control or your birth control failed. It can be used up to 120 hours (five days) after unprotected sex to prevent pregnancy. There are two main types of emergency contraception:

1. Emergency contraceptive pills (ECPs): Depending on the type of ECPs, you can use them within three days or within five days after unprotected sex to prevent pregnancy

2. The copper T IUD can be used to prevent pregnancy up to five days after unprotected sex.

Advantages of emergency contraception

- Does not require the consent of the female's partner
- Is safe and effective in preventing pregnancy after unprotected sex
- Some are available over the counter

Drawbacks of emergency contraception

- Not as effective as some other types of birth control
- Requires a clinic visit and a prescription in some cases
- Does not work if you are already pregnant
- May cause side effects like nausea (anti-nausea medication might help with this), vomiting, stomach pain, and headaches
- Does not protect against sexually transmitted infections

Effectiveness:

Emergency Contraceptive Pills:

Plan B One-Step, Next Choice One Dose, My Way and Levonorgestrel Tablets: Seven out of eight women who would have gotten pregnant will not become pregnant after taking these pills.

ella: Six or seven out of every 100 women who would have gotten pregnant will not become pregnant after taking ella.

IUD:

The copper T IUD is the most effect emergency contraceptive method. Out of 1,000 women who use this method, only one will get pregnant.

How do I get emergency contraception?

ECPs are available at some pharmacies. Women and men of all ages can get emergency contraceptive pills besides ella without a prescription. You may want to check that your local pharmacy carries ECPs before making a trip there.

Women of all ages need a prescription for ella. Contact your healthcare provider to get a prescription. Many family planning clinics dispense emergency contraceptive pills and offer IUDs as a birth control option.

BIRTH CONTROL IN DEPTH:
FEMALE STERILIZATION

Permanently prevents pregnancy, will not prevent the sexual spread of Zika.

Female sterilization is a choice for women who are certain they do not want to get pregnant. While it will prevent pregnancy, it will not protect against the sexual spread of Zika. Some important CDC information on this birth control method is included below.

What is female sterilization?

Female sterilization permanently prevents women from becoming pregnant. There are two different procedures to achieve this goal, tubal ligation and tubal implants. They both work by blocking the fallopian tubes (tubes that lead from women's ovaries into the uterus or womb) so that sperm cannot meet with and fertilize an egg.

Because these methods cannot be undone, they are only recommended for women who are sure they never want to have a baby or who do not want to have more children.

Tubal ligation: The fallopian tubes are cut, sealed, or tied. With this method, very tiny cuts (called incisions) are made in the abdomen or belly. This is also known as having "tubes tied" or tubal ligation. Surgical sterilization works to prevent pregnancy right away.

Tubal implant: A very small spring-like coil is placed into each fallopian tube. The coils cause scar tissue to form in the tubes, thereby blocking the tubes. This method does not involve cuts or incisions. Instead, a healthcare provider uses a thin tube to thread the small coils through the vagina and uterus into the fallopian tubes, where the coils will stay.

With the tubal implant, it will take up to three months for the scar tissue to fully block the tubes. So, it is important to use a back-up type of birth control (like a condom or the birth control shot) until your health care provider says it is not needed. You will go back to the health center or office for an exam and be checked to make sure the coils are in the right place and the tubes are blocked. This may require a special type of X-ray where dye is placed into the uterus to make sure the tubes are blocked.

Advantages of female sterilization

- Safe and highly effective approach to preventing pregnancy
- Lasts a lifetime, so no need to worry about birth control again
- Quick recovery
- No significant long-term side effects
- Your male partner doesn't have to know about it or do anything different.

Drawbacks of female sterilization

- Does not protect against sexually transmitted infections (STIs), including HIV
- Some risk of infection, pain, or bleeding
- Very rarely, the tubes can grow back together. When this happens there is a risk for pregnancy. In some cases, this leads to tubal or ectopic pregnancy—when the

pregnancy happens in the fallopian tubes, which is a life-threatening condition.

- Some women later change their mind and wish they could have a child or additional children.

Effectiveness

- Out of 100 women who have a sterilization procedure each year, fewer than one may become pregnant.

How do I get it?

Female sterilization is a relatively simple outpatient surgery done in a health center, doctor's office, or hospital. It can be performed under local or general anesthesia, depending on the method used to perform sterilization. You will go home the same day.

To search for a family planning center near you, go to www.hhs.gov/opa

BIRTH CONTROL IN DEPTH: MALE STERILIZATION

Will prevent pregnancy, will not prevent the sexual spread of Zika.

Like female sterilization, male sterilization will prevent pregnancy, but it will not prevent the sexual spread of Zika. Important CDC information on this topic is included below:

What is male sterilization?

Male sterilization, or vasectomy, is a procedure performed on a man that will permanently keep him from being able to get a woman pregnant.

Vasectomy is an outpatient procedure done under local anesthesia. After the local anesthesia is injected, the health care provider then makes tiny cuts (incisions) in the scrotum, the sac that holds the testes or "balls." The vas deferens—two tubes that carry sperm to the penis—are then cut, tied, or blocked.

Some men receive a no-scalpel vasectomy where, instead of cutting the skin of the scrotum, very tiny holes are made. The tubes that carry sperm are pulled through the holes and tied off and cut. A no-scalpel vasectomy does not require stitches.

After a vasectomy, a man will still produce semen, the fluid that comes out of his penis when he has sex. A man will need to return to his health provider after about three months to be tested to make sure there are no more sperm in his semen. It takes about three months to clear the sperm out of the system. A man should use another type of birth control (like a condom) until his healthcare provider tells him there are no longer any sperm in his semen.

There may be surgery available to reverse a vasectomy, but men should consider the procedure permanent. Before a vasectomy, men can also freeze their sperm for future use if they choose.

Advantages

- The man's partner doesn't have to know about it or do anything different.
- Lifts the contraceptive burden from the woman
- Safe and highly effective approach to preventing pregnancy
- Lasts a lifetime, so no need to worry about birth control again
- The procedure is simple to do and usually involves only a little bit of discomfort

- Quick recovery time after the procedure
- Most cost-effective of all birth control methods

Drawbacks

- Provides no protection against sexually transmitted infections (STIs), including HIV
- Requires a visit to a clinic or medical office
- Risk of swelling, bruising, and tenderness for a short time after the procedure
- Very rarely, the tubes that carry sperm can grow back together. When this happens there is a risk of pregnancy.
- Some men, or their partners, later change their minds and wish they could have a child or additional children.

Effectiveness in Preventing Pregnancy

Out of 100 women each year whose partner has had a vasectomy, fewer than one may get pregnant.

Where can I get a vasectomy?

A vasectomy can be done in a medical office or clinic. It is an outpatient procedure, so a man can go home the same day.

While not all family planning clinics perform vasectomies, your local family planning clinic may be able to tell you where vasectomy is available in your area. To find a family planning center near you, use OPA's clinic locator at www.hhs.gov/opa.

PREGNANCY AND EXPOSURE TO A ZIKA-PRONE LOCATION

If you are pregnant and are considering traveling to a location with Zika, consider again. The CDC currently recommends against travel to locations with active Zika transmission. If you must go, or you live in an area with Zika, it would be wise to follow the CDC's advice for travelers to Zika-prone areas. CDC advice for travel to Mexico is excerpted below, although it should provide valuable guidance to anyone living in an area with Zika, or those traveling to another country which is also experiencing Zika:

What can travelers do to prevent Zika?

There is no vaccine or medicine for Zika. Travelers can protect themselves by preventing mosquito bites:

- Cover exposed skin by wearing long-sleeved shirts and long pants.
- Use EPA-registered insect repellents containing DEET, picaridin, oil of lemon eucalyptus (OLE, also called para-menthane-diol [PMD]), or IR3535. Always use as directed.
  - Pregnant and breastfeeding women can use all EPA-registered insect repellents, including DEET, according to the product label.
  - Most repellents, including DEET, can be used on children older than two months. (OLE should not be used on children younger than three years.)
- Use permethrin-treated clothing and gear (such as boots, pants, socks, and tents). You can buy pre-treated clothing and gear or treat them yourself.
- Stay in places with air conditioning and window and door screens to keep mosquitoes outside.
- Sleep under a mosquito bed net if air-conditioned or screened rooms are not available or if sleeping outdoors.

- Mosquito netting can be used to cover babies younger than two months old in carriers, strollers, or cribs to protect them from mosquito bites.

Because Zika can be sexually transmitted, if you have sex (vaginal, anal, or oral) while traveling, you should use condoms.

After travel

Many people infected with Zika virus do not feel sick. If a mosquito bites an infected person while the virus is still in that person's blood, it can spread the virus by biting another person. **Even if they do not feel sick, travelers returning to the United States from Mexico should take steps to prevent mosquito bites for three weeks so that they do not spread Zika to uninfected mosquitoes.**

Travelers returning from Mexico who have a pregnant partner should either use condoms or not have sex for the rest of the pregnancy.

People who have traveled to Mexico should use condoms for at least eight weeks after travel to protect their sex partners. Men who have Zika symptoms or are diagnosed with Zika should use condoms for at least six months after symptoms start; women with symptoms should use condoms for at least eight weeks after symptoms start.

Travelers who are thinking about pregnancy should talk with their health care provider. Men who have traveled to Mexico should wait at least eight weeks after travel before trying to conceive or at least six months after symptoms start if they develop symptoms of Zika. Women who have traveled to Mexico should wait at least eight weeks after travel before trying to get pregnant, or at least eight weeks after symptoms start if they develop symptoms.

If you feel sick and think you may have Zika

- Talk to your doctor if you develop a fever with a rash, joint pain, or red eyes. Tell him or her about your travel.
- Take acetaminophen (paracetamol) to relieve fever and pain. Do not take aspirin, products containing aspirin, or other nonsteroidal anti-inflammatory drugs, such as ibuprofen.
- Get lots of rest and drink plenty of liquids.

If you are pregnant

Talk to a doctor or other health care provider after your trip, **even if you don't feel sick**. Pregnant travelers returning from Mexico or who have had possible sexual exposure should be offered testing for Zika virus infection.

- If you develop a fever with a rash, joint pain, or red eyes, talk to your doctor immediately and tell him or her about your travel or possible sexual exposure.
- If you do not have symptoms, testing should be offered if you see a health care provider, up to twelve weeks after you return from travel or your last possible sexual exposure.

7

Microcephaly

OVERVIEW AND RISK FROM ZIKA

Any parent will agree that there is nothing more important than their child's life and well-being. The scariest effects of Zika are perhaps its effects on babies, who are sometimes born with smaller-than-normal heads and retarded brain development, a condition known as microcephaly. Researchers are still trying to figure out the odds that a mother with Zika will give birth to a baby with microcephaly. Studies have come to different conclusions, with the odds ranging from a possible 1 percent[21] risk to a much more shocking 29 percent risk.[22] The CDC has identified the major symptoms, causes, and side effects of microcephaly. Adapted below, this section covers the information you need to know about this serious condition.

WHAT IS MICROCEPHALY?

Microcephaly is a condition where a baby's head is much smaller than expected. During pregnancy, a baby's head grows because the baby's brain grows.

Microcephaly can occur because a baby's brain has not developed properly during pregnancy or has stopped growing after birth, which results in a smaller head size.

Microcephaly can be an isolated condition, meaning that it can occur with no other major birth defects, or it can occur in combination with other major birth defects.

What is severe microcephaly?

Severe microcephaly is a more serious, extreme form of this condition where a baby's head is much smaller than expected. Severe microcephaly can result because a baby's brain has not developed properly during pregnancy, or the brain started to develop correctly and then was damaged at some point during pregnancy.

Other problems

Babies with microcephaly can have a range of other problems, depending on how severe their microcephaly is. Microcephaly has been linked with the following problems:

- Seizures
- Developmental delay, such as problems with speech or other developmental milestones (like sitting, standing, and walking)
- Intellectual disability (decreased ability to learn and function in daily life)
- Problems with movement and balance
- Feeding problems, such as difficulty swallowing
- Hearing loss
- Vision problems

These problems can range from mild to severe and are often lifelong. Because the baby's brain is small and underdeveloped, babies with severe microcephaly can have more of these problems, or have more difficulty with them, than babies with milder microcephaly. Severe microcephaly also can be life-threatening. Because it is difficult to predict at birth what problems a baby will have from microcephaly, babies with microcephaly often need close follow-up through regular check-ups with a healthcare provider to monitor their growth and development.

Occurrence

Microcephaly is not a common condition. State birth defects tracking systems have estimated that microcephaly ranges from two babies per 10,000 live births to about twelve babies per 10,000 live births in the United States.

Causes and Risk Factors

The causes of microcephaly in most babies are unknown. Some babies have microcephaly because of changes in their genes. Other causes of microcephaly, including severe microcephaly, can include the following exposures during pregnancy:

- Certain infections during pregnancy, such as rubella, toxoplasmosis, or cytomegalovirus.
- Severe malnutrition, meaning a lack of nutrients or not getting enough food
- Exposure to harmful substances, such as alcohol, certain drugs, or toxic chemicals
- Interruption of the blood supply to the baby's brain during development

Some babies with microcephaly have been reported among mothers who were infected with Zika virus while pregnant. CDC scientists announced that enough evidence has accumulated to conclude that Zika virus infection during pregnancy is a cause of microcephaly and other severe fetal brain defects.

CDC continues to study birth defects, such as microcephaly, and how to prevent them. If you are pregnant or thinking about becoming pregnant, talk with your doctor about ways to increase your chances of having a healthy baby.

Diagnosis

Microcephaly can be diagnosed during pregnancy or after the baby is born.

During pregnancy

During pregnancy, microcephaly can sometimes be diagnosed with an ultrasound test (which creates pictures of the body). To see microcephaly during pregnancy, the ultrasound test should be done late in the second trimester or early in the third trimester.

AFTER THE BABY IS BORN

To diagnose microcephaly after birth, a healthcare provider will measure the distance around a newborn baby's head, also called the head circumference, during a physical exam. The provider then compares this measurement to population standards by sex and age. Microcephaly is defined as a head circumference measurement that is smaller than a certain value for babies of the same age and sex. This measurement value for microcephaly is usually less than two standard deviations (SDs) below the average. The measurement value also may be designated as less than the third percentile. This means the baby's head is extremely small compared to babies of the same age and sex.

Head circumference growth charts for newborns, infants, and children up to age twenty years in the United States can be found on CDC's growth charts website. Head circumference growth charts based on gestational age at birth (in other words, how far along the pregnancy was at the time of delivery) are also available from INTERGROWTH 21st. CDC recommends that health care providers use the WHO growth charts to monitor growth for infants and children ages zero to two years of age in the United States.

Often, healthcare providers should take the head circumference measurement when the newborn baby is at least twenty-four hours old. This helps make sure that compression due to delivery through the birth canal has resolved. If the healthcare provider suspects the baby has microcephaly, he or she can request one or more tests to help confirm the diagnosis. For example, special tests like a CT scan or an MRI can provide critical information on the structure of the baby's brain that can help determine if the newborn baby had an infection during pregnancy. They also can help the healthcare provider look for other problems that might be present.

TREATMENTS

Microcephaly is a lifelong condition. There is no known cure or standard treatment for microcephaly. Because microcephaly can range from mild to severe, treatment options can range as well. Babies with mild microcephaly often don't experience any other problems besides small head size. These babies will need routine check-ups to monitor their growth and development.

For more severe microcephaly, babies will need care and treatment focused on managing their other health problems (mentioned above). Developmental services early in life will often help babies with microcephaly to improve and maximize their physical and intellectual abilities. These services, known as early intervention, can include speech, occupational, and physical therapies. Sometimes medications also are needed to treat seizures or other symptoms.

ENDING A PREGNANCY

If you have been exposed to Zika and are pregnant, you may be considering having an abortion. Depending on many factors including the stage of the pregnancy, your personal preferences, and local laws, this procedure may be an option. State laws vary widely in this regard, with some states prohibiting abortion after viability, and other states allowing later termination of a pregnancy. Further restrictions may exist for women under the age of eighteen.

If you have contracted Zika and are in a foreign country, getting an abortion may be exceptionally difficult. Most countries in Latin America have strict rules limiting or prohibiting the procedure altogether. Abortion is a serious procedure that requires professional medical advice. If you want to learn more, be sure to talk to a healthcare professional who can assist you.

8

Guillain-Barré Syndrome

OVERVIEW AND CORRELATION WITH ZIKA

Although microcephaly has attracted headlines as the most notable negative effect of Zika, the virus is also associated with Guillain-Barré syndrome, which can cause paralysis.

The central question about Zika and GBS—how much does Zika increase the odds of getting GBS?—is currently unanswerable. That's because we simply don't know enough about Guillain-Barré. That's right: it is such a rare condition that there is precious little previous information on the syndrome, giving new researchers little to go on. Annalisa Merelli of Quartz writes, ". . . many things remain unknown, including the likelihood of occurrence. We don't have much data to understand whether anything makes developing GBS more likely—partially because we don't have much data about GBS, full stop."[23]

While we truly do not know how much getting Zika increases the odds of getting GBS, anecdotal evidence suggests that only a relatively small minority of Zika cases progress to full-blown Guillain-Barré. Interestingly, Zika-stricken adults appear much more susceptible to GBS than children.

The National Institute of Neurological Disorders and Stroke has a large amount of information about this serious condition, some of which has been excerpted below.

WHAT IS GUILLAIN-BARRÉ SYNDROME?

Guillain-Barré syndrome is a disorder in which the body's immune system attacks part of the peripheral nervous system. The first symptoms of this disorder include varying degrees of weakness or tingling sensations in the legs. In many instances the symmetrical weakness and abnormal sensations spread to the arms and upper body. These symptoms can increase in intensity until certain muscles cannot be used at all and, when severe, the person is almost totally paralyzed. In these cases the disorder is life threatening—potentially interfering with breathing and, at times, with blood pressure or heart rate—and is considered a medical emergency. Such an individual is often put on a ventilator to assist with breathing and is watched closely for problems such as an abnormal heartbeat, infections, blood clots, and high or low blood pressure. Most individuals, however, have good recovery from even the most severe cases of Guillain-Barré syndrome, although some continue to have a certain degree of weakness.

Guillain-Barré syndrome can affect anybody. It can strike at any age and both sexes are equally prone to the disorder. The syndrome is rare, however, afflicting only about one person in 100,000. Usually Guillain-Barré occurs a few days or weeks after the patient has had symptoms of a respiratory or gastrointestinal viral infection. Occasionally surgery will trigger the syndrome. Recently, some countries worldwide have reported an increased incidence of GBS following infection with the Zika virus. In rare instances, vaccinations may increase the risk of GBS.

After the first clinical manifestations of the disease, the symptoms can progress over the course of hours, days, or weeks. Most people reach the stage of greatest weakness within the first two weeks after symptoms appear, and by the third week of the illness, 90 percent of all patients are at their weakest.

WHAT CAUSES GUILLAIN-BARRÉ SYNDROME?

No one yet knows why Guillain-Barré—which is not contagious—strikes some people and not others. Nor does anyone know exactly what sets the disease in motion.

What scientists do know is that the body's immune system begins to attack the body itself, causing what is known as an auto-immune disease. Usually the cells of the immune system attack only foreign material and invading organisms. In Guillain-Barré syndrome, however, the immune system starts to destroy the myelin sheath that surrounds the axons of many peripheral nerves, or even the axons themselves (axons are long, thin exten-sions of the nerve cells; they carry nerve signals). The myelin sheath surrounding the axon speeds up the transmission of nerve signals and allows the transmission of signals over long distances.

In diseases in which the peripheral nerves' myelin sheaths are injured or degraded, the nerves cannot transmit signals efficiently. That is why the muscles begin to lose their ability to respond to the brain's commands, commands that must be car-ried through the nerve network. The brain also receives fewer sensory signals from the rest of the body, resulting in an inabil-ity to feel textures, heat, pain, and other sensations. Alternately, the brain may receive inappropriate signals that result in tingling, "crawling-skin," or painful sensations. Because the signals to and from the arms and legs must travel the longest distances they are most vulnerable to interruption. Therefore, muscle weakness and tingling sensations usually first appear in the hands and feet and progress upwards.

When Guillain-Barré is preceded by a viral or bacterial infection, it is possible that the virus has changed the nature of cells in the nervous system so that the immune system treats them as foreign cells. It is also possible that the virus makes the immune system itself less discriminating about what cells it recognizes as its own, allowing some of the immune cells, such as certain kinds of lymphocytes and macrophages, to attack the myelin. Sensitized T lymphocytes cooperate with B lymphocytes to produce antibodies against components of the myelin sheath and may contribute to destruction of the myelin. In two forms of GBS, axons are attacked by antibodies against the bacteria *campylobacter jejuni*, which reacts with proteins of the peripheral nerves. Acute motor axonal neuropathy is particularly common in Chinese children. Scientists are investigating these and other possibilities to find why the immune system goes awry in Guillain-Barré syndrome and other autoimmune diseases. The cause and course of Guillain-Barré syndrome is an active area of neurological investigation, incorporating the cooperative efforts of neurological scientists, immunologists, and virologists.

HOW IS GUILLAIN-BARRÉ SYNDROME DIAGNOSED?

Guillain-Barré is called a syndrome rather than a disease because it is not clear that a specific disease-causing agent is involved. A syndrome is a medical condition characterized by a collection of symptoms (what the patient feels) and signs (what a doctor can observe or measure). The signs and symptoms of the syndrome can be quite varied, so doctors may, on rare occasions, find it difficult to diagnose Guillain-Barré in its earliest stages.

Several disorders have symptoms similar to those found in Guillain-Barré, so doctors examine and question patients carefully before making a diagnosis. Collectively, the signs and symptoms form a certain pattern that helps doctors differentiate Guillain-Barré from other disorders. For example, physicians will note whether the symptoms appear on both sides of the body (most common in Guillain-Barré) and the quickness with which the symptoms appear (in other disorders, muscle weakness may progress over months rather than days or weeks). In Guillain-Barré, reflexes such as knee jerks are usually lost. Because the signals traveling along the nerve are slower, a nerve conduction velocity (NCV) test can give a doctor clues to aid the diagnosis. In Guillain-Barré patients, the cerebrospinal fluid that bathes the spinal cord and brain contains more protein than usual. Therefore a physician may decide to perform a spinal tap, a procedure in which a needle is inserted into the patient's lower back and a small amount of cerebrospinal fluid from the spinal column is withdrawn for study.

HOW IS GUILLAIN-BARRÉ SYNDROME TREATED?

There is no known cure for Guillain-Barré syndrome. However, there are therapies that lessen the severity of the illness and accelerate the recovery in most patients. There are also a number of ways to treat the complications of the disease.

Currently, plasma exchange (also called plasmapheresis) and high-dose immunoglobulin therapy are used. Both of them are equally effective, but immunoglobulin is easier to administer. Plasma exchange is a method by which whole blood is removed from the body and processed so that the red and white blood cells are separated from the plasma, or liquid portion of the blood. The blood cells are then returned to the patient without the plasma, which the body quickly replaces. Scientists still don't know exactly why plasma exchange works, but the technique seems to reduce the severity and duration of the Guillain-Barré episode.

This may be because plasmapheresis can remove antibodies and other immune cell-derived factors that could contribute to nerve damage.

In high-dose immunoglobulin therapy, doctors give intravenous injections of the proteins that, in small quantities, the immune system uses naturally to attack invading organisms. Investigators have found that giving high doses of these immunoglobulins, derived from a pool of thousands of normal donors, to Guillain-Barré patients can lessen the immune attack on the nervous system. Investigators don't know why or how this works, although several hypotheses have been proposed.

The use of steroid hormones has also been tried as a way to reduce the severity of Guillain-Barré, but controlled clinical trials have demonstrated that this treatment not only is not effective but may even have a deleterious effect on the disease.

The most critical part of the treatment for this syndrome consists of keeping the patient's body functioning during recovery of the nervous system. This can sometimes require placing the patient on mechanical ventilatory assistance, a heart monitor, or other machines that assist body function. The need for this sophisticated machinery is one reason why Guillain-Barré syndrome patients are usually treated in hospitals, often in an intensive care ward. In the hospital, doctors can also look for and treat the many problems that can afflict any paralyzed patient—complications such as pneumonia or bed sores.

Often, even before recovery begins, caregivers may be instructed to manually move the patient's limbs to help keep the muscles flexible and strong and to prevent venous sludging (the buildup of red blood cells in veins, which could lead to reduced blood flow) in the limbs, which could result in deep vein thrombosis. Later, as the patient begins to recover limb control, physical therapy begins. Carefully planned clinical trials of new and experimental therapies are the key to improving the treatment of patients with Guillain-Barré syndrome. Such clinical trials begin with the research of basic and clinical scientists who, working with clinicians, identify new approaches to treating patients with the disease.

WHAT IS THE LONG-TERM OUTLOOK FOR THOSE WITH GUILLAIN-BARRÉ SYNDROME?

Guillain-Barré syndrome can be a devastating disorder because of its sudden and unexpected onset. In addition, recovery is not necessarily quick. As noted above, patients usually reach the point of greatest weakness or paralysis days or weeks after the first symptoms occur. Symptoms then stabilize at this level for a period of days, weeks, or, sometimes, months. The recovery period may be as little as a few weeks or as long as a few years. About 30 percent of those with Guillain-Barré still have a residual weakness after three years. About 3 percent may suffer a relapse of muscle weakness and tingling sensations many years after the initial attack.

Guillain-Barré syndrome patients face not only physical difficulties, but emotionally painful periods as well. It is often extremely difficult for patients to adjust to sudden paralysis and dependence on others for help with routine daily activities. Patients sometimes need psychological counseling to help them adapt.

WHAT RESEARCH IS BEING DONE?

Scientists are concentrating on finding new treatments and refining existing ones. Scientists are also looking at the workings of the immune system to find which cells are responsible for beginning and carrying out the attack on the nervous system.

The fact that so many cases of Guillain-Barré begin after a viral or bacterial infection suggests that certain characteristics of some viruses and bacteria may activate the immune system inappropriately. Investigators are searching for those characteristics. Certain proteins or peptides in viruses and bacteria may be the same as those found in myelin, and the generation of antibodies to neutralize the invading viruses or bacteria could trigger the attack on the myelin sheath. As noted previously, neurological scientists, immunologists, virologists, and pharmacologists are all working collaboratively to learn how to prevent this disorder and to make better therapies available when it strikes.

9

Zika's Effect on the World

ZIKA'S EFFECTS ON POLITICS

Zika is not just a global health problem; it is a political one as well. Zika has exacerbated tensions between Venezuela and Colombia, neighboring countries in Latin America, who have pointed fingers at each other over their countries' respective handling of the crisis. It has also entered the United States presidential campaigns in a big way.

Long regional rivals, the Venezuela and Colombia have seen their relationship continue to be pressured by the epidemic. Venezuela has refused to coordinate medical care or even talk to Colombia about the issue. Colombian officials have also accused Venezuela of deliberately underreporting Zika cases.[24] Venezuela, which is in the midst of a major political and economic crisis, lacks adequate supplies of medicine, birth control, and even food, and it is unclear how much the country could to do to stem the crisis even if it had a better relationship with Colombia.

In the United States, Zika was a political flashpoint in the presidential race between Hillary Clinton and Donald Trump.

On March 18, 2016, Hillary Clinton argued forcefully for more funding for the Zika epidemic. "Zika is real. It's dangerous. It's already reached the United States. We need to act now to protect people, especially pregnant women. There are smart, achievable things we could be doing right now, and there's no time to waste. So we need Congress to act. We need citizens to demand action."[25]

In August of 2016, Republican nominee Donald Trump offered his opinion on Zika, optimistically arguing the governor of Florida would be able to keep the virus under control, saying, "You have a great governor who's doing a fantastic job—Rick Scott—on the Zika. And it's a problem. It's a big problem. But I watch and I see. And I see what they're doing with the spraying and everything else. And I think he's doing a fantastic job and he's letting everyone know exactly what the problem is and how to get rid of it. He's going to have it under control. He probably already does."[26]

Some observers were disappointed that Trump had few specifics on Zika, although Trump's Miami-Dade campaign vice-chair called the issue "insignificant,"[27] arguing, "We have so many other issues that are more important than this." During a campaign stop in Miami, Clinton said, "I disagree with those who say that Zika is an insignificant issue. My opponent in this race, his campaign officials have said that, and I think that it does a grave disservice." During the same appearance, she said, "This is an epidemic that will only grow." She added, "We don't want to wake up in a year and read so many more stories about babies like the little girl who just died in Houston."[28] Clinton was referring to a young baby born with microcephaly who died due to complications related to her condition.

Zika divided the two campaigns, who seemed to disagree on the seriousness of the issue. While Clinton offered more specific solutions regarding how she would deal with the epidemic as president, as of mid-August Trump and his campaign had downplayed the risk, arguing that there were other serious issues facing the nation. As more Americans continue to learn about Zika, we can expect more politicians at all levels to discuss the issue. Indeed, if past is prologue, we can also expect more partisan rancor over this issue.

RELIGION, BIRTH CONTROL, AND ZIKA

The Zika crisis has brought many Latin American countries' policies on birth control and abortion to the forefront of an international discussion about religious belief and reproductive health. Much of Latin America is heavily Catholic, and the Vatican has long considered the use of birth control to be a sin. Although birth control is widely available in many locations, the Church's strict teachings against it have led many in these heavily Catholic nations to forgo its use.

Abortion is an even more controversial topic. The procedure is banned in Nicaragua, El Salvador, and the Dominican Republic, and is only legal when necessary to save the life of the mother in Guatemala, Haiti, Honduras, Paraguay, Suriname, and Venezuela. Most other Latin American countries also have strict controls as well. Conservative attitudes about birth control and abortion have come into conflict with the health challenge that the Zika epidemic presents. Crucial to this debate is the Catholic Church, whose moral teachings are the foundation of many local laws on abortion and contraception.

Although the pope has always been an important and revered figure in Latin America, Pope Francis is particularly influential as he was born in Argentina. Thus, many wondered about his opinion on the Zika epidemic, and particularly whether the use of birth control or abortion to prevent pregnancy would be permissible.

Pope Francis, who was born in Buenos Aires, was asked about the issue in early 2016. He responded first by reiterating the Catholic Church's position on abortion, disappointing those who thought the Church might soften its stance given the Zika epidemic. He said, "Abortion is not the lesser of two evils. It is a crime. It is to throw someone out in order to save another. That's what the Mafia does. It is a crime, an absolute evil."[29] Yet while he was unyielding in his disapproval of abortion, he did seem to suggest that, given the Zika outbreak, birth control could be permissible, saying, "Don't confuse the evil of avoiding pregnancy by itself with abortion." He added, "Avoiding pregnancy is not an absolute evil." Pope Francis also encouraged development of a vaccine, saying, "I would also urge doctors to do their utmost to find vaccines against these two mosquitoes that carry this disease. This needs to be worked on."

Given the fervent belief of many Catholics in South America, these statements were welcomed by many who felt it might encourage the use of birth control and help prevent the spread of Zika. At the same time, the pope's unyielding stance on abortion also provoked controversy amongst those who believe the procedure should be more easily obtainable in the region. In short, while his statements marked a slight concession from traditional Catholic doctrine, they did not mark a significant shift away from existing Church teachings. The debate over birth control, abortion, and religion is likely to continue long into the future.

TIMELINE OF IMPORTANT EVENTS

1947: Zika first discovered, in a Ugandan monkey.

1952: The first cases of Zika in humans are identified in Uganda and Tanzania.[30]

1953–2006: Zika continues to exist and spread, primarily in Africa and Asia. Infections are rare, outbreaks seemingly do not occur, and the virus is widely regarded as a minor threat.

2007: There is a Zika outbreak on Yap Island, in the Federated States of Micronesia. This is the first known major outbreak in recorded history.

2008: A US scientist infects his wife with Zika after contracting the virus during field work in Senegal. This is likely the first documented case of the sexual transmission of the virus.[31]

2013–2014: In October, Zika outbreaks strike French Polynesia, New Caledonia, the Cook Islands, and Easter Island.[32] Increased cases of Guillain-Barré appear.

2015: From February to April 29, around 7,000 cases of a mystery virus are reported in northeastern Brazil. Authorities did not test for Zika, as the virus was not suspected to be in Brazil.[33]

On May 7, the National Reference Laboratory of Brazil reports that Zika is spreading in their country.[34]

Although first detected in Brazil, Zika quickly spreads across Latin America, reaching Colombia, Panama, Mexico, Surname, Venezuela and other countries in the region.

In November, American Samoa reports its first case of locally acquired Zika, making this the first time the virus has spread in portions of the US

On December 31, Puerto Rico reports its first case of locally acquired Zika.

2016: On January 15, the CDC advises pregnant women to avoid travel to areas hit by Zika.

Pope Francis tacitly endorses the temporary use of birth control as a means to stop the spread of Zika.

On April 6, the Obama administration reroutes $589 million, most of which was originally earmarked to fight ebola, towards fighting Zika.

On June 28, the Senate fails to agree on a bill to fight Zika, halting progress towards more funding to fight the virus.

By August, nearly 500 New Yorkers have caught Zika, five of them through sex.[35]

On August 1, the CDC announces that the virus has begun spreading in the US mainland for the first time, and advises pregnant women to avoid Wynwood, a neighborhood of Miami, Florida, struck by the virus.

The Surgeon General of the United States has estimated that by the end of 2016, 25 percent of Puerto Ricans—approximately 875,000 people—will contract Zika.

10

How You Can Help

OVERVIEW

Facing a threat like Zika, it can be hard to know what to do. This is an international disease infecting millions of people. Can a single person really make a difference? The answer is yes. By taking action in your local community, and reaching out to legislators and government decision-makers, you can help create and implement change.

ORGANIZING IN YOUR AREA

Perhaps the most important step you can take is spreading knowledge about Zika while organizing to make sure you and the members of your community are protected.

Zika is likely to continue to spread across parts of the United States. Even if it hasn't struck your community, you'll want to be prepared, so informing your neighbors and community members about the virus is key. Even if they've heard of the virus, they may not know the symptoms, the correct precautions, or what to do if they're infected. With this guidebook and the latest updates from organizations like the CDC, you'll be well informed and ready to help educate others.

Consider talking to your local school boards about holding meetings for parents and students at your local elementary school. Consider contacting local preschools, churches, or other organizations that are likely to have large numbers of expectant mothers in their ranks. As pregnant women and their unborn children are most vulnerable to Zika, targeting this group as part of your outreach effort is key to mitigating the effects of the disease.

Organizing local volunteer or outdoors groups to help in the fight against mosquitoes is also extremely important. As mosquitoes are the primary way the virus spreads, taking extra care to eliminate their habitats and control their numbers is crucial to mitigating the spread of Zika. Although community-wide efforts are best, the fight against mosquitoes starts with you. Check the areas around your house or apartment for standing water, and make sure your neighbors are also aware of the threat mosquitoes face. Even if you do not feel threatened by the disease, a mosquito on your property may go on to infect a pregnant woman in another part of town. When it comes to Zika and mosquitoes, we're truly all in this together.

There are many valuable resources that can help you organize and spread the word about Zika. Meetup.com, a platform for creating groups of like-minded people, is one powerful tool. It enables you to create groups, send email notifications, and help rally interested people to your cause. You might also consider creating a Facebook page or Twitter list of interested community members. You'll be able to share ideas and work to organize other concerned citizens in your area.

Whether you decide to create an online group, work with local charities and church groups, or simply decide to discuss the Zika virus with your friends and community members, be sure to responsibly spread the word about the challenges Zika poses. Remember, while Zika does present some serious risks, the effects of the virus are usually minimal. To get the message across effectively, it's important to neither exaggerate nor understate the risks. Focus on finding solutions for those who are most vulnerable to the virus—pregnant women—while seriously but calmly stating the generally lesser risks that other community members face.

CALL YOUR LEGISLATOR

Although there is much that you can do at a local level, an epidemic like Zika deserves a national response. The signature bill that was designed to fight Zika is currently being held up in Congress. Be sure to call your legislator or senator to push for the passage of a bill that will focus on eliminating and mitigating Zika within the United States. Although political gridlock is a common aspect of today's US political system, the stakes are simply too high for continued inaction. While both political parties have tried to shift the blame onto one another, Americans have been contracting the virus. One child has even died as a result of it. Although political posturing may be a good election strategy, it is a poor way to address public health threats to our nation.

Given that Zika can be spread through sexual contact, we must also be proactive in increasing the availability of birth control and correct education around its use. Since the Zika virus inflicts perhaps its most severe damage on infants, it is crucial that birth control and safe sex options like condoms are available for pregnant mothers, women planning on becoming pregnant, and women who have a partner infected with Zika.

Finally, ensuring that scientific research to combat the disease is adequately funded and pursued at a national level is crucial to the fight against Zika. Without the knowledge of Zika's weaknesses and how it may be overcome, we will be unable to truly stop the spread of this disease. While work on a vaccine is ongoing, we must be sure we are able to devote the resources necessary to continue funding this important research.

Regrettably, we cannot be certain that efforts to fight Zika will be fully funded. We still don't know the exact correlation between Zika and Guillain-Barré syndrome, throwing uncertainty on an already stressful and unpredictable epidemic. We also still don't know the odds that a mother infected with Zika will give birth to a baby with microcephaly. Estimates vary widely, with percentages from 1 percent to 29 percent being debated. More research will enable us to truly understand Zika and, hopefully, prevent more children from being born with microcephaly.

Although the effects of Zika are not as severe as some other diseases, it is important that we adequately understand the risks posed by the virus. Right now, there is too much about Zika that we simply do not know.

Whether it is passing a bill to address the Zika epidemic, ensuring there is access to birth control, or funding scientific research on the virus, all of these steps require action by legislators at the national level. Call, email, or write to your representatives in Congress requesting action on this important health problem that may soon be at risk of infecting millions of Americans.

Congress

To contact your senators, visit www.senate.gov/senators/contact. To find your representative, visit www.house.gov/representatives/find.

The president

To call the president, use this phone number:
Comments: 202–456–1111
TTY/TTD
Comments: 202–456–6213

11

Additional Resources

Interested in taking action? Want to learn more? Use this list of resources to discover the latest information on Zika, contact professionals, or figure out ways you can get involved.

HEALTH ORGANIZATIONS

Centers for Disease Control
1600 Clifton Road Atlanta, GA 30329–4027 USA
800-CDC-INFO (800–232–4636), TTY: 888–232–6348
www.cdc.gov

CDC Zika Website
This CDC website contains up-to-date information on Zika and the threats it poses around the world.
www.cdc.gov/zika

World Health Organization
World Health Organization
Avenue Appia 20
1211 Geneva 27
Switzerland
Telephone: + 41 22 791 21 11
Facsimile (fax): + 41 22 791 31 11
www.who.int

WHO Zika Homepage
This WHO website contains a wealth of information on the current spread of Zika around the world.
http://www.who.int/emergencies/zika-virus/en/

WHO Zika Situation Report
The World Health Organization puts out a weekly Zika situation report that details the current spread of the virus, what health organizations are doing to fight the virus, and other relevant information.
www.who.int/emergencies/zika-virus/situation-report/en

VECTOR CONTROL ORGANIZATIONS
Vector control organizations are dedicated to spreading awareness of vector-borne diseases and helping prevent their spread. They have a wealth of knowledge of local threats that are spreading diseases like Zika. Although the naming may seem strange, "vector" simply refers to insects and animals that spread disease. Thus, in the case of Zika, the "vector" that spreads Zika are mosquitoes.

American Mosquito Control Organization
www.mosquito.org

Association of Structural Pest Control Regulatory Officials
www.aspcro.org

Mosquito Research Foundation
www.mosquitoresearch.org

National Pesticide Information Center
National Pesticide Information Center

Oregon State University
310 Weniger Hall
Corvallis, OR 97331–6502
Phone: 800–858–7378
E-mail: npic@ace.orst.edu
Hours: 8:00 a.m. to 12:00 p.m. PST, Monday—Friday
http://npic.orst.edu/

STATE VECTOR CONTROL ASSOCIATIONS

Mosquito and Vector Control Organization of California
http://www.mvcac.org/

Florida Mosquito Control Association
www.floridamosquito.org

Louisiana Mosquito Control Association
www.lmca.us

Michigan Mosquito Control Association
www.mimosq.org

South Carolina Department of Health and Environmental Control
www.scdhec.gov

Texas Mosquito Control Association
www.texasmosquito.org

Utah Mosquito Abatement Association
www.umaa.org

Virginia Mosquito Control Association
www.mosquito-va.org

FIND YOUR LOCAL VECTOR CONTROL CONTACT

Vector control agencies coordinate programs to eliminate mosquitoes and other public health threats that can spread disease.

Visit www.npic.orst.edu/vecmlr.html to find your local vector control contact.

The mosquito and vector control association of California has compiled a list of many vector control organizations on their website. The list can be found at: www.mvcac.org/resources/mosquito-and-vector-control-associations-and-organizations

PODCASTS

CNN Podcasts on Zika
A collection of helpful CNN podcasts relating to the Zika Virus.
http://podcast.cnn.com/explore/Zika-virus.

CDC Podcasts
A collection of CDC podcasts, including information on mosquito bites and Zika.
https://www2c.cdc.gov/podcasts/

DOCUMENTARIES

Love in the Time of Zika
An informative and heartbreaking documentary on the tough choices facing women infected with Zika. Available on multiple websites, including:
http://documentaryheaven.com/love-in-time-of-zika/

Spillover—Zika, Ebola & Beyond.
This PBS documentary discusses the Zika and ebola epidemics, providing viewers with a balanced view of the situation. http://www.pbs.org/show/spillover-zika-ebola-beyond/

EVENTS

January is National Birth Defect Prevention Month. Find out more about this important annual event on the CDC website. www.cdc.gov/ncbddd/birthdefects/prevention-month.html

About the Author

Alexander Webb is the founder of *Take Risks Be Happy*, an online magazine for creatives, entrepreneurs, and travelers. He was shortlisted for the 2015 Bracken Bower Prize and was a contributing writer for National Geographic's *The Civil War: A Traveler's Guide*. His is the co-author of *Shock Markets*, published by the Financial Times Press, and released in Chinese translation in 2015. He currently lives in California.

Laura D. Kramer, PhD, FASTMH (Fellow of the American Society of Tropical Medicine and Hygiene), has been studying the ecology, epidemiology, and evolution of mosquito-borne viruses for more than forty years. She is currently director of the Arbovirus Laboratories of the Wadsworth Center, New York State Department of Health, and professor of biomedical sciences, School of Public Health, State University of New York at Albany. Her lab conducts surveillance for and research on vector-borne viruses in New York State. Dr. Kramer also is a virology moderator for the Program for Monitoring Emerging Diseases (ProMED-mail).

References

1   Chen, Lin H. MD, Hamer, Davidson H. MD. "Zika Virus: Rapid Spread in the Western Hemisphere." *Annals of Internal Medicine.* May 3, 2016. http://annals.org/article.aspx?articleid=2486362

2   Ibid.

3   England, Charlotte. "A quarter of the population of Puerto Rico are expected to get the Zika virus." *The Independent.* August 13, 2016. http://www.independent.co.uk/news/world/zika-virus-puerto-rico-public-health-emergency-us-obama-administration-a7188776.html

4   Carroll, Linda. Sarmiento, Samuel, MD. "'Striking' Results from Early Zika Vaccine Trial." NBC News. August 4, 2016. http://www.nbcnews.com/storyline/zika-virus-outbreak/striking-results-early-zika-vaccine-trial-n623016

5   Press Release: "Expansion of Oxitec's Vector Control Solution in Brazil Attacking Source of Zika Virus and Dengue Fever after Positive Program Results." Oxitec, January 19, 2016. http://www.oxitec.com/oxitec-vector-control-solution-in-brazil-attacking-source-of-zika-virus/.

6   Monitoring Microcephaly Cases in Brazil. August 11, 2016. http://portalsaude.saude.gov.br/images/pdf/2016/agosto/17/Informe-Epidemiol–gico-n—39–SE-32-2016–16ago2016-19h10.pdf. http://www.oxitec.com/oxitec-vector-control-solution-in-brazil-attacking-source-of-zika-virus/.

7   Rosenbloom, Stephanie. "Where Will Americans Travel in 2015?" *The New York Times.* January 6, 2015. http://www.nytimes.com/2015/01/11/travel/where-will-americans-travel-in-2015-.html

8   "Casos Confirmados de Enfermedad por virus del Zika", *Semana epidemiológica 31 del 2016.* August 15, 2016. http://www.epidemiologia.salud.gob.mx/doctos/avisos/2016/zika/DGE_ZIKA_CASOS_SEM31_2016.pdf

9   England, Charlotte. "A quarter of the population of Puerto Rico are expected to get the Zika virus." *The Independent.* August 13, 2016. http://www.independent.co.uk/news/world/zika-virus-puerto-rico-public-health-emergency-us-obama-administration-a7188776.html

10 Ulmer, Alexandra. "Venezuelan women seek sterilizations as crisis sours child-rearing." Reuters. August 3, 2016. http://www.reuters.com/article/us-venezuela-sterilizations-idUSKCN10E1NK

11 Aizenman, Nurith. Sullivan, Becky. "Venezuela Won't Talk to Colombia About Zika—And That's A Problem." *NPR.* February 23, 2016. http://www.npr.org/sections/goatsandsoda/2016/02/23/467803305/venezuela-wont-talk-to-colombia-about-zika-and-thats-a-problem

12 Casciano, Edgard Antonio. "Brazil's engagement in the fight against the Zika virus epidemic." *Ekathimerini.com* February 29, 2016. http://www.ekathimerini.com/206459/article/ekathimerini/comment/brazils-engagement-in-the-fight-against-the-zika-virus-epidemic

13 Carroll, Linda. Sarmiento, Samuel, MD. "'Striking' Results from Early Zika Vaccine Trial." NBC News. August 4, 2016. http://www.nbcnews.com/storyline/zika-virus-outbreak/striking-results-early-zika-vaccine-trial-n623016

14 Zhou, Winnie. Blanchard, Ben. Fernandez, Clarence. "WHO chief going to the Olympics, says Zika risk low." MSN, July 29, 2016. http://www.msn.com/en-us/sports/olympics/who-chief-going-to-the-olympics-says-zika-risk-low/ar-BBv1c2x

15 Mansuy, Jean Michael. Dutertre, Marine. Mengelle, Catherine. Fourcade, Camille. Marchou, Bruno. Delobel, Pierre. Izopet, Jacques. Martin-Blondel, Guillaume. "Zika virus: high infectious viral load in semen, a new sexually transmitted pathogen?" *The Lancet.* Vol. 16, No. 4. P405. April 2016.

16 Zika found to remain in sperm for record six months. BBC News, August 12, 2016. http://www.bbc.com/news/health-37057934

17 McConnell, Mitch. "Senate Democrats Block Support for Veterans, Anti-Zika Efforts." "Remarks delivered on Senate floor, June 28, 2016. http://www.republicanleader.senate.gov/newsroom/remarks/senate-democrats-block-support-for-veterans-anti-zika-efforts

18 Herszenhorn, David M. "Zika Bill is Blocked By Senate Democrats Upset Over Provisions." "*New York Times,* June 28, 2016. http://www.nytimes.com/2016/06/29/us/politics/congress-zika-funding.html

19 Fox, Maggie. "Zika Virus Fight: White House Shifts Ebola Cash, Blames Congress." NBC News. April 6, 2016. http://www.nbcnews.com/storyline/zika-virus-outbreak/white-house-shift-ebola-funds-zika-fight-n551631

20 Bichell,RaeEllen."HowBesttoTestForZikaVirus?NPR."March10,2016. http://www.npr.org/sections/health-shots/2016/03/10/469549176/ how-best-to-test-for-zika-virus

21 Johansson, Michael A. Ph.D,, Mier-y-Teran-Romero, Luis, Ph.D., Reefhuis, Jennita, Ph.D., Gilboa, Suzanne M. Ph.D., Hills, Susan L. Ph.D. "Zika and the Risk of Microcephaly." *The New England Journal of Medicine.* July 7, 2016. http://www.nejm.org/doi/full/10.1056/ NEJMp1605367?query=featured_zika

22 McNeil, Donald G. Jr. Louis, Catherine Saint. "Two Studies Strengthen Links Between the Zika Virus and Birth Defects." *New York Times.* March 4, 2016. http://www.nytimes.com/2016/03/ 05/health/zika-virus-microcephaly-fetus-birth-defects.html?

23 Merelli, Annalisa. "Why we can't say how likely Zika is to leave you temporarily paralyzed." *Quartz.* June 10, 2016. http://qz.com/703282/why-we-cant-say-how-likely-zika-is-to-leave-you-temporarily-paralyzed/

24 Aizenman, Nurith. Sullivan, Becky. "Venezuela Won't Talk to Colombia About Zika—And That's A Problem." NPR. February 23, 2016. http://www.npr.org/sections/goatsandsoda/2016/02/23/467803305/ venezuela-wont-talk-to-colombia-about-zika-and-thats-a-problem

25 Clinton, Hillary. The time to take action against Zika is now. *Medium.* March 18, 2016. https://medium.com/hillary-for-america/the-time-to-take-action-against-zika-is-now-aa40f325a3f7#. jdailgw03.

26 Diamond, Jeremy. "Trump punts to Florida governor on Zika." *CNN.* August 3, 2016. http://www.cnn.com/2016/08/03/politics/ zika-donald-trump-rick-scott-election-2016

27 Ibid.

28 "VERBATIM: Clinton attacks Trump on Zika." *Reuters TV.* August 9, 2016. www.reuters.tv/v/DKf/2016/08/09/verbatim-clinton-attacks-trump-on-zika

29 Full text of Pope Francis' in-flight interview from Mexico to Rome. *Catholic News Agency.* February 18, 2016. http://www.catholicnewsagency.com/news/full-text-of-pope-francis-in-flight-interview-from-mexico-to-rome-85821/

30 "The history of Zika virus." World Health Organization. http:// www.who.int/emergencies/zika-virus/timeline/en/

31 Kindhauser, Mary Kay. Allen, Thomas. Frank, Veronika. Santhana, Ravi Shankar. Dye, Christopher. "Zika: the origin and spread of a mosquito-borne virus." *Bulletin of the World Health Organization.* February 9, 2016. http://www.who.int/bulletin/online_first/16–171082.pdf

32 Ibid.

33 Ibid.

34 Ibid.

35 Gonen, Yoav. Almost "500 New Yorkers have tested positive for Zika virus." *New York Post.* August 16, 2016. http://nypost.com/2016/08/16/almost-500-new-yorkers-have-tested-positive-for-zika-virus